ARTICULATION THERAPY
AND CONSONANT DRILL BOOK

ARTICULATION THERAPY

AND

CONSONANT DRILL BOOK

By

SIDNEY GODA, Ph.D.

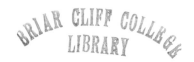

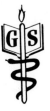

GRUNE & STRATTON
New York and London

LB
3454
.Y58

For Adelle, who has learned that children need time before they fully master the phonological dimensions of the language. For Bruce, Randi, and William, who have provided longitudinal evidence of this growth and of the inconsistency of consonant mastery on the way to full acquisition. For Chris, David, Ross, Kathy, Michael, and many other children with articulation errors, who have provided clinical evidence that consonant errors are rarely consistent. For the students in speech pathology at the University of North Carolina in Chapel Hill and Greensboro, who listened and asked meaningful questions during the summers when these ideas were presented. And for Dr. Campton Bell, of the University of Denver, who taught me very early the importance of keeping your eyes on the stars and your feet firmly on the ground.

Preface

The materials in this book are primarily intended for persons with articulation disorders, by far the most common type of speech disorder among children and adults alike. Regardless of setting, whether public school, private school, hospital, or private practice, the caseload of the speech pathologist is predominantly made up of defective speakers with articulation disorders. The articulation disorder may be of functional etiology and the only type of speech disorder, or it may be of organic etiology and associated with a voice disorder such as in individuals who have cleft palates. Children with brain damage, whether minimal or as extensive as in cerebral palsy, children with peripheral or central hearing difficulties, children with aphasia, and children with mental retardation may all have disorders of articulation in addition to other kinds of speech disorders. Adults, as a result of illness, traumatic injury, or cerebral vascular accident, may also produce consonant phonemes incorrectly.

The book has two principal divisions, the drill materials and the rationale for articulation therapy.

The drill materials have been selected very carefully from Thorndike and Lorge's *Teacher's Word Book of 30,000 Words* (1944). Except for certain voicing and other phonemic contrasts, all words are at or below the fourth grade reading level of this source. Drill material is arranged according to age of phonemic mastery by normal-speaking children. Words are divided according to word length, since one-syllable words are more easily produced than polysyllabic words by persons with articulation difficulty. In addition, the drill materials are divided by parts of speech so that the speaker will be able to move immediately from the isolated word level to the grammatical use of speech in two-, three-, and four-word phrases and structurally complete sentences.

The therapy approach is based on normative data concerning the way children master articulation, and on research findings which show conclusively that articulation errors are usually inconsistent and therefore that there are words in which production is already correct. Valuable time is saved if training begins immediately with those words in which production is already correct and is gradually extended to those words which contain phonetic contexts in which production is incorrect. Variables

vii

affecting correctness and inconsistency of production are discussed together with implications for therapy procedures and methods. Attention is called to the function of the breath stream and what speakers do to arrest and release the breath stream for speaking.

The rationale for speech therapy, discussed in some detail, presents a point of view which could result in effective results over relatively short periods of time. We all recognize the fact that the number of speech and hearing clinicians in schools and hospitals is inadequate for the large numbers of persons in need of speech and hearing therapy. As a result, the clinician needs to carry a heavy caseload and maintain a waiting list for children who cannot be accommodated. With the approach described here, more children could be helped and thus the size of caseloads and numbers on waiting lists could be reduced significantly.

This drill book should lighten the task of the speech pathologist, who frequently needs to spend considerable time developing word lists and organizing speech materials from many diverse sources. At present, the clinician who teaches children at several different schools needs to utilize many diverse sources—books, journals, manuscripts—in order to compile suitable drill materials. A single source book containing suitable speech drills can easily be taken from school to school; numerous volumes and manuscripts can be very clumsy and tedious. Time devoted to speech therapy will be more effectively utilized when a single source is used, since time will not be lost in the changing, arranging, and shifting about of different materials. While the speech clinician in hospitals, clinics, and private practice is not necessarily faced with the task of transporting different materials, he or she needs to spend countless hours organizing appropriate speech materials from different sources. A single source book can lighten the task of this group as well.

The drill material could also be used by the teacher of the early elementary grades to facilitate the growth of consonant mastery. The sequence in language arts consists of listening, speaking, reading, and writing, in that order (Olson, 1959). The child understands spoken symbols before he uses them for speaking. He needs to be able to use spoken symbols at a relatively high level before he can handle written symbols. Materials can be selected for the purpose of developing listening skills and auditory discrimination, both vital and necessary before the child is able to read or write with any degree of proficiency. The reading teacher can use these word lists to develop a reading vocabulary and teach word attack. The remedial reading teacher can use them to develop phonic ability with children who are not reading up to grade level or up to potential.

Adults with dysarthria following cerebral vascular accident or traumatic injury frequently have articulation errors involving consonant sounds because of cranial nerve involvement. They can relearn how to produce phonemes acceptably in single-word responses but may have considerable difficulty in production of phonemes in polysyllabic words. The organization of this book should be valuable for the dysarthric patient.

Textbooks in the field of speech pathology are frequently theoretical without specific application. But the practicing clinician needs material to use directly in his handling of patients. Therefore, many clinicians develop what might be called an eclectic approach to articulation therapy. In so doing, they feel they are avoiding error because they are borrowing from many different persons or sources and because they have been told that this "works." Unfortunately, many do not question the logic or rationale of eclecticism nor can they fit their material into a comprehensive scheme. We need to carefully explore our approaches to articulation therapy, to question them and our methods continuously. We may find that our methods are not entirely effective, and that in fact the defective speaker may experience emotional harm as a result of our approach and our lack of recognition of particular needs. We need to be constantly critical of what we are doing and honest in our appraisal of ourselves and our results.

The particular approach presented here is offered with considerable humility and with the full realization that several basic issues are far from being clarified: the etiology of the articulation disorders, particularly the so-called functional disorders, and the factors in the retraining program which lead to correction or prevent correction. In time, these issues may be elucidated by research and clinical effort. Meanwhile, the author feels that his approach has a sound rationale and can effect results for those who wish to try and adapt it to their own needs.

SIDNEY GODA

Contents

PREFACE vii

1. ARRANGEMENT OF DRILL MATERIALS 1
   Source of Material 1
   Age of Phonemic Mastery 1
   Position Classification Abandoned 2
   Principal Parts of Speech 6
   Phonemic Classification 10

2. DRILL MATERIALS 14
   Consonants I 14
   Consonants II 20
   Consonants III 34
   Consonants IV 41
   Consonants V 56
   Consonants VI 60
   Blends I 66
   Blends II 78
   Blends III 80
   Consonants and Blends 84
   Phonemic Contrasts 90

3. TREATMENT FOR ARTICULATION DISORDER 102
   Assessment of Articulation 102
   Articulation Treatment 105
   Whole Word Method of Assessment and Treatment . . . 113

4. FURTHER PROCEDURES IN ARTICULATION THERAPY ADAPTED
   TO AGE LEVEL 143
   Preschool Children 144
   Early Elementary School Age Children 151
   Older Children and Adults 153
   Individual Therapy versus Group Therapy 154
   Length and Frequency of Speech Therapy Sessions . . . 155
   Parental Involvement 155

REFERENCES 157
INDEX 159

1. Arrangement of Drill Materials

Speech problems in children and adults may involve phonological, grammatical, and lexical dimensions (Winitz, 1966). The speech materials in this book are for persons with poor articulation who are producing consonant sounds incorrectly, the phonological aspect. Persons with the lone speech disorder of defective articulation involving errors in consonant production can constitute as much as 95 per cent of the caseload of the speech and hearing clinician.

SOURCE OF MATERIAL

The word lists contained in this book are all at or below the fourth grade reading level in Thorndike and Lorge's *Teacher's Word Book of 30,000 Words* (1944), with the exception of voicing and other contrast lists. They are organized to provide practice drill for persons with articulation difficulty of either functional or organic origin.

Many words used with great frequency today were relatively unknown when Thorndike and Lorge's book was published. These words can be added at the teacher or clinician's discretion. It will be very obvious that such words as *television, missile, atomic, astronaut, lunar, orbit,* etc., are missing from the word lists. Further it will be obvious that some words included in this book are in fact beyond the fourth grade reading level. These words can be utilized for the high school child or adult. Words can be selected judiciously from the available lists for the child in the second and third grades. Pictures to elicit the word can be used for the nonreader or poorer reader. The appropriate vocabulary for the individual child should determine the words which are selected for drill. The child's interests, age, and linguistic level should determine the vocabulary items. Proper names are not included in the drill lists with the exception of the contrast lists. The words are organized so that the other two aspects, involving grammar and lexicon, can figure prominently and early in speech training. A later section will describe the organization.

AGE OF PHONEMIC MASTERY

The order of the sound presentation coincides with the latest developmental data concerning age of mastery of the different consonant types

(Templin, 1957). The earliest learned sounds appear to be those which require the least modification of the breath stream, and the sounds which are learned later apparently involve greater modifications of the breath stream. Earliest learned sounds are the nasals, which involve a continuation of the breath stream through the nasal cavity. Plosives are also learned early because the modification of the breath stream is relatively uncomplicated, stopping momentarily and releasing again. Other consonant types, fricatives and affricates or combinations, are learned last. They require a more subtle modification of the breath stream. Consonants are mastered first as singles before they are mastered as blends. Mastery of two consonant blends precedes that of three consonant blends.

The nasal consonants appear first in the drill book, followed by plosives, semivowels, fricatives, and combinations or affricates in that order. Materials for the /r/ follow, and separate word lists are devoted to three different /r/ sounds as described by Curtis and Hardy (1959): stressed vocalic, unstressed vocalic, and consonant glide. Materials for blends appear last in the drill section, with double consonant blends coming before triple consonant blends. There are no materials either for vowels, with the exception of the vocalic [r] and vocalic [l], or for diphthongs because elementary school age children rarely misarticulate these. Seventy-five per cent of the three-year-old children in Templin's study had mastered production of all vowels and diphthongs.

POSITIONAL CLASSIFICATION ABANDONED

The positional classification of a consonant (with the exception of the vocalic /r/, which must be treated as a vowel for teaching purposes) as initial, medial, or final, as described in the textbooks in the field of speech pathology (Berry and Eisenson, 1956; Johnson et al., 1967; Van Riper, 1965; Van Riper and Irwin, 1958) and suggested as a basis for articulation training in drill books (Fairbank, 1960; Schoolfield, 1951), is abandoned here in favor of classification of the consonant according to its function within a syllable. Taking precedence from Stetson's analyses (1951) and McDonald's very recent applications (1964A), a consonant is classified according to its function within the syllable, either serving as the arresting or releasing element of the syllable. Classification of a sound as medial obscures this function, since sounds occurring within bisyllabic and polysyllabic words either serve as arresting elements of one syllable or releasing elements of another. Most important, classifying a consonant according to its function within the syllable centers attention on the breath stream and the modifications placed upon the breath stream for the overlaid function of speaking. With this scheme, the child thinks about what he does when speaking, a concept which can be important in the correction of articulation errors, as we shall see in a later section. The child attends to what he does with the breath stream for correct production of the consonant phoneme, as contrasted with changes previously imposed on the breath stream for incorrect production.

The number of syllables contained in a word will affect the ease of production. The task of consonant production is obviously easiest when the consonant arrests or releases words which contain one syllable only. When the sound occurs in the second or subsequent syllables of a polysyllabic word, the articulation requirements are more difficult, involving a more complicated motor act with increased retention span. Even within one syllable words, the number of individual sounds will affect the ease of articulation of the consonant. The child newly learning the sound will find the production easiest in words having only one additional sound besides the defective sound. In addition to the function of the consonant, each separate word list is further divided according to the number of syllables and phonetic elements within the word.

Releasing Consonant

One-syllable words containing two phonetic elements, the consonant element as the releasing element and one other phoneme, are the first words in the list in which the consonant releases the syllable. The remaining words of one syllable have more phonetic elements following the consonant as a releasing element. Bisyllabic and polysyllabic words in which the consonant releases the first syllable appear after words of one syllable. Then come drill words of more than one syllable, in which the consonant functions to release the second syllable while attention is still paid to the number of elements following the releasing consonant. Words of three or more syllables, in which the consonant releases the third syllable, follow. The few polysyllabic words in which the consonant releases syllables beyond the third appear last on the list.

Arresting Consonant

The same scheme as listed above is followed for the arresting consonant, except that the consonant functions to arrest the syllable. The first words listed are one-syllable words with the consonant as the arresting element and with only one phonetic element prior to the consonant. One-syllable words with more phonetic elements contiguous to the arresting consonant follow. Then come words of two or more syllables in which the consonant arrests the first syllable, and words of two or more syllables in which the consonant arrests the second syllable. The last words are polysyllabic words in which the consonant arrests the third, fourth, or subsequent syllables.

The principal word lists are for drill on consonants which have one function only, that of arresting or releasing the breath stream. Some lists contain drill words in which the consonant functions in a multifaceted manner to both arrest and release the breath stream, to arrest the breath stream more than once, or to release the breath stream more than once. Consonant production will generally be easiest in those words which require the consonant to have only a single function. The initial blend lists contain words with only a single blend. Some lists contain words with more than one consonant blend.

One cannot always be sure with words of two or more consonants whether the consonant arrests the syllable or releases the syllable which follows. Opinions differ concerning appropriate syllable division. Curtis and Hardy (1959) give an example in their study of misarticulation of /r/, mentioning that the word *apron* may be spoken in two ways: with the combination /pr/ produced as a consonant blend which initiates the second syllable or divided so that the /p/ and /r/ belong to different syllables with different functions, the /p/ arresting the first syllable and the /r/ releasing the second syllable. They make a separate analysis of these "intersyllabic /r/ contexts" in which there is "real uncertainty concerning appropriate division of a word into syllables." Blends involving /s/ and /l/ present similar difficulties in syllabication.

There is no ultimate source to use in the solution of this problem of syllable division. It will be apparent that some words in the drill book have a syllable division which is different from that of the Merriam Webster. The article "Divisions in Respelled Pronunciation" in *Webster's Third New International Dictionary*, unabridged (1968, page 47a), recognizes the difficulties inherent in any syllabic division, and that because there are "extremes of opinion with regard to syllable boundaries, whatever course a dictionary adopts will meet with some opposition." The *Webster's New World Dictionary* states (1964, page xx):

To decide where one syllable ends and another begins, however, is a matter of such difficulty that linguistic science is still unable to provide a simple formula for syllable division in English. The separation of syllables in this and similar books is merely a graphic convenience intended to help printers to be consistent. Its virtues are esthetic, not linguistic. . . . we have represented to us a system which is neither logical in itself nor based in any degree on the ascertained characteristics of our language.

Webster's New International Dictionary, Second Edition, unabridged (1955), discusses the difficulty of deciding in the word *apple* whether the second syllable begins after, before, or within the /p/. Reference is made to Stetson, who says that syllable division depends on the rate of speech and that any increase in speech will carry the consonant into the movement of the second syllable. Nonetheless, this work lays down ten very complex rules of orthography which are also applied to speaking. *Webster's Third New International*, unabridged, becomes very critical of one of these rules, the practice of treating a single consonant as being in the following syllable when preceded by a long stressed vowel or an unstressed vowel, and as being in the same syllable with a preceding short stressed vowel. If this rule is followed, the word *apron* is divided so that the /p/ releases the second syllable, but in the word *tablet* the /b/ arrests the first syllable and the /l/ releases the second.

The thesis of this author is that of not viewing phonemes as static, fixed entities and thus it expresses strong disagreement with a fixed positional system of error location. The author suggests the need for flexibility of consonant function dependent on the preference of the individual speaker and the phonetic context. This need becomes particularly apparent in production of phonemes in isolated words as compared with their production in connected speech. As we shall see later, the consonant function in an isolated word becomes different when that word is included as a unit in a larger phonetic context. Therapeutic results become possible rather quickly if this relative view of consonant function is accepted by both clinician and defective speaker very early. Many examples are given later of enhancement of results from therapy because of changing consonant function of the error phoneme.

The author has used his own judgment, based on many years of academic and clinical experience in listening to normal speakers, in deciding on syllable division. The author feels that the syllable division presented here is essentially that of the normal speaker. However, there may well be different opinions among users of the book, in which case persons can knowingly change the syllable division of words in the book because of the individual preference or to hasten results in articulation training.

Certain consistencies will become apparent to users of the book. The viewpoint of the author is that consonants generally change their function when morphemes are added to root words. The final consonant in the root word merges to release the second syllable. The /m/ in *charm, tame*, and *come* arrests these one-syllable words but releases the second syllable with addition of morphemes, as in *charming, charmer, taming, tamer*. In words with double letters, such as *apple, oppose*, and *apply*, the consonant will be viewed as releasing the second syllable. When two or more consonants which may be used together to begin a syllable come between two vowels, as in *apron, tablet*, and *abrupt*, they will generally be joined together as a blend to release the second syllable.

The ultimate goal of articulation therapy is correct production of the error phoneme in conversational speech. Necessary subgoals prior to complete mastery of the sound are correct production in isolated words and in words which are part of phrases or sentences extended from the word level. The grammatical aspect of spoken language is an important dimension with extended utterances. Syntax, the arrangements or relationships of words to one another, is the chief ingredient of grammar. The materials in this book are arranged so that longer utterances involving phrases and sentences can be generated easily from the isolated word lists.

PRINCIPAL PARTS OF SPEECH

The drill words are separated further into the three principal parts of speech: nouns, verbs, and adjectives. Fries' study (1952) of the running speech of adults reveals that these three parts of speech made up a large part of his recorded material, 81 per cent of a thousand recorded words. A fourth group of words, designated as "Other," includes the other parts of speech which make up the remaining 19 per cent. Fries designates two classes of words for the "Other" parts of speech used here, adverbs and so-called function words. If a word serves as more than one part of speech, it may be listed more than once under the appropriate parts of speech. The isolated words in a specific list can be readily combined with each other and with other words to form two-, three-, and four-word phrase units. The phrase units can be further extended to form structurally complete simple sentences. Some few examples follow of the many phrase units of varying length which can be constructed very easily.

TWO-WORD UNITS

Units of two words in length can be constructed easily with nouns by prefacing each noun with the articles or function words *a*, *an*, and *the* (Fries, 1952). Possessive pronouns *my*, *his*, *her*, *our*, *your*, and *their* and adjectives for color, quantity, shape, or quality can also be combined with nouns to form phrase units of two words in length. Verbs can form two-word units when prefaced with the personal pronouns *I*, *we*, *they*, and *you* and plural nouns. The personal pronouns *he* and *she* and singular nouns may also be combined with verbs to form two-word units, but attention must be paid to the change in verb endings, which will usually involve the addition of the morphemes /-s/ or /-es/. In some instances nouns and verbs from the same list may be joined together. Adjectives can form two-word units when paired with appropriate nouns, as mentioned earlier in discussing nouns.

THREE-WORD UNITS

Units of three words in length can be formed by joining like parts of speech with the connective words *and* and *or*. Verbs can be used to form three-word units in imperative sentences, which are structurally complete without a subject. For example, with the verb list where /p/ releases the initial syllable, the following commands could be uttered: *Pass the book, Pat the table, Pour the milk, Push the wagon*, etc. Three-word phrases could be formed with adjectives by prefacing the two-word unit of adjective and noun with the articles *a, or, an*, and *the*, or the possessive pronouns *my, your, his, her, our*, or *their*. Prepositions listed in the "Other" category may be used to form three-word units by combining with nouns and articles or appropriate adjectives. Such prepositions as *in, on, under, with, down, up, after*, and *to* may be used to form such phrases as *in my house, in your pocket, on Daddy's car, under our porch, with my friend, down the street, down the road, up the steps, to the movie, to my school*, etc.

FOUR-WORD AND LARGER UNITS

Phrase units greater in length than three words can be formed by combining an appropriate noun with two adjectives joined by a connective word or by combining a personal pronoun with two verbs joined by a connective word. For example, the following four- and five-word phrase units could be formed with some of the verbs and adjectives found in the /p/ release list: *the poor but happy boy, the pale and pink flower, I push and you pull, We push and pull, They paint and I paste*. Prepositional phrases made up of more than three words will result from addition of appropriate adjectives.

STRUCTURALLY COMPLETE SIMPLE SENTENCES

Structurally complete simple sentences can be formed by extending the four-word phrase units or any smaller units. Structurally complete simple sentences could be formed by completing the following open-ended phrases with a noun: *I see the _____, I don't see the _____, I saw the _____, I will see the _____, I have the _____, I like the _____, I want the _____, I found the _____*, etc. The carrier phrase *Say the word* or *I say the word* will form structurally complete sentences if prefaced before each word in a list. If the /l/ is the error phoneme and sentence units are needed for drill, the carrier phrases, *I like the color* or *I don't like the color* could preface each color word depending upon the choices of the child. The carrier phrases *I like the food* or *I don't like the food* could preface the names of foods for sentence drills for either the /l/ or /f/ phoneme. The carrier phrases *I like* *the toy, I want the toy, I see the toy,* or *I have the toy* could preface the names of toys for sentence drills for the /t/, /w/, /s/, /d/, and /h/ phonemes.

Favorite toys could provide a topic through which further sentence drills may be developed. For example, the question could be asked: *Do you like the toy horn? Yes, I like the horn,* or the negative transformation *I don't like the horn* would be the response, depending on the child's preference. When the child expresses a preference for the toy, the following dialogue could ensue: *What do you do with the toy horn? I blow it. Who else can blow the horn? Nobody else,* or *My sister can,* or *My mother can,* or *My teacher can. When do you blow the horn? At a party, In a parade, In a band,* etc.

Articles of clothes could furnish an excellent topic for sentence drill for children working on correct production of plosives in sentences.

TEACHER: Mary, I see you are wearing something new.
MARY: Yes, I have a new hat and coat.
TEACHER: They are a pretty color.
MARY: I always like red. Red is a bright color.
TEACHER: John, I like the color of your shirt.
JOHN: I don't. It's black, and black is too dark.
TEACHER: How many like the color red? How many like the color black? How many liked the color red?
SUSIE: I counted two.
TEACHER: And how many liked the color black?
SUSIE: The same number, two.
TEACHER: Do you like black?
SUSIE: I have a black dress which I like very much.
TEACHER: Tell me about your black dress.

Discussions of seasons of the year or holidays could provide excellent topics for children working on a variety of different sounds. If we continue with drill on plosives:

TEACHER: What time of the year do you like best?
JOHN: I like winter best.
TEACHER: Tell me why.
JOHN: I can go skiing on weekends.
TEACHER: That sounds like fun. Where do you go?
(John answers from his own experiences with pertinent questions from everyone.)
TEACHER: Who likes summer best?
SUSIE: I do.
TEACHER: What can you do?
SUSIE: We go on picnics, hikes, and go swimming in pools and lakes.

Discussion of costs of items could provide topics for children working on affricates or fricatives.

TEACHER: I saw some beautiful shoes for sale at Gimbel's. Who wants to ask me something?
JOHN: How much were they?
TEACHER: Black shoes were $10.00, but white shoes were more.
JOHN: How much were the white shoes?
TEACHER: They were $12.00. Are white shoes worth more than black shoes?
JOHN: No, the white shoes are too much.

Noun catagories of animals can be prefaced with appropriate carrier phrases to form complete sentences for drill on /z/: *The tiger is in the zoo, The zebra is in the zoo, The elephant is in the zoo, My dog is not in the zoo.*

In summary, let us take several single nouns from the /p/ arrest list and illustrate how linguistic units containing the error phoneme may be extended. Initially the child reads or repeats the words *cap, cup, rope,* and *ship.* The articles *a* and *the* as well as possessive pronouns *my* and *you* are combined with each word, resulting in phrase units of two words *my cup, my rope, my ship, a cup, a rope, a ship.* Following mastering of phonetic production with two-word phrase units, three-word units can be formed through the use of the connective word *and* to yield the phrases *cap and cup, cup and rope, rope and ship, ship and cap.* The adjectives *large, big, small,* and *little* can be used with the nouns to form the phrases *a large ship, a small ship, a big ship, a little ship, a large cup, a small cup,* etc. Other adjectives may be added to form phrase units larger in length than three words. Finally, structurally complete units can be formed through extending the phrases and use of the verbs *is, see,* and *have.* The sentences formed are: *The cup is large, The cup is big, The ship is large, The ship is big,* etc.; *I see the cup, I see the ship; I have the cup, I have the ship.* Adjectives may be used with the last groups of sentences to form more complicated linguistic units resulting in the sentences *I see the large ship, I see the big ship.*

Connective words or conjunctions *and, or, but,* and *if* can be used with structurally complete simple sentences to form all kinds of sentences. The simple sentences can be expanded: *I see the cup and I see the fish. I have the cup, but I do not have the rope. If the rope is too small, I will not see it.*

The following verbs can be drilled on for mastery of /t/: *take, tell, tie, touch.* Two-word phrases can develop through combining the verbs with the various personal pronouns or plural nouns: *I take, I tell, I tie, I touch,* etc. Three-word units develop from joining two verbs by the connectives *and* and *or* to form the units: *Take and tell, Tell and tie, Tie or touch, Touch or take*, etc. Three word phrases will result by combining other appropriate words with the verbs: *I tell you, I tell him, I tell mother, I tell teacher, I tie my shoes, I tie your shoes, I take this, You take that, You touch your nose, You touch the book.* The game "Simon says" can perhaps be introduced at this point, with particular attention to correct production of the phoneme /t/ each time the verb *touch* is spoken. Other pronouns and singular nouns can be combined with verbs, but changes need to be made in the verb endings: *He tells, She takes, He ties, Baby touches, Father touches, Teacher takes,* etc. Compound sentences will be formed by joining simple sentences with *and: I tell father, and father tells mother, You touch your nose, and baby touches his toes.*

The adjective *good* and *sick* may be combined with appropriate nouns if drill material is needed for the plosives /g/ and /k/ to form the phrases: *a good girl, a good guy, a good dog, a good cat, a sick girl, a sick dog, a sick cat.* Longer sentences will emerge with use of the verbs *is* or *see: I see the sick girl, The dog is sick,* etc. Using the connective *but*, the following compound sentences emerge: *The dog is sick, but the cat is not sick, The dog is big but the cat is little.*

While these kinds of sentence drills are not appropriate for older children or adults, suitable materials can be developed from the drill lists in a manner similar to that utilized in extending the words into sentence drills for children. Early drill material for adults can, as for children, begin with production of single words. Phrases can be developed from nouns by pairing the nouns with articles, prepositions, adjectives, or other nouns as has been discussed before. These kinds of simple drills are particularly useful with stutterers when quantity of material is significant. Adults with voice problems will learn to produce a pleasant voice in material made up of single words and phrases, but hoarseness or harshness may result with longer materials. When the stutterer develops easier speech in materials involving single words and phrases, longer sentences can be introduced in the manner outlined previously, through carrier phrases, open-ended sentences, and conversation involving particular interests. The person with a voice quality disorder will need to remain at the word and phrase levels until the quality is acceptable before longer units are introduced.

When the child is producing the phoneme correctly in all kinds of sentences covering many different topics of conversation, he is ready for carry-over in which he attends to production of the sound in spontaneous speech.

PHONEMIC CLASSIFICATION

This drill book is concerned with the phonemic status of the sounds which occur in the English language only, without comparing or considering the phonemic systems in other languages. The phonemes of the English language will be considered and contrasted with each other. These phonemes will be defined only in terms of their differences from the other phonemes in our language. As such, the phoneme discussed and then involved in particular word lists will be denoted by slash marks. However, when there are two or three clearly distinct types of sounds all representing the same phoneme, these different types are allophones and are denoted by brackets (Gleason, 1961; Hockett, 1958). It is interesting to note that Gleason considers an articulation error involving a lisp to be the use of an "incorrect allophone of a single phoneme /s/" (Gleason, 1961, page 343).

Three allophones will be subsumed under /r/: stressed vocalic [ɝ], unstressed vocalic [ɚ], and consonant glide [r]. Two allophones will be subsumed under /l/: the vocalic [l̩] and semivowel [l].

MANNER, PLACEMENT, AND VOICING

While the consonants will be grouped according to developmental data from Templin's study, consonant sounds will be described further through the use of the three dimensions employed by Fairbanks (1960) and Johnson et al. (1967): manner, placement, and voicing. The first dimension, that of manner, allows for the grouping of sounds according to type on the basis of the kinds and extent of change which are imposed on the breath stream in order to produce the different types of consonant phonemes. With the exceptions of glides and semivowels, consonant phonemes introduce changes in the breath stream by diverting, impeding, or restricting the stream. When an individual can successfully handle these different modifications, he is able to produce all consonants as single sounds. The semivowels, classified as consonants III in the drill materials which follow, interfere only slightly with the passage of the breath stream by minimal interference or obstruction. Glides involve no change as such on the breath stream. Movement with mouth shaping is the significant feature of the glides.

The materials are divided according to the apparent complexity of breath stream modification, with the initial sounds being those which require the least modification and later sounds being those which require relatively greater modification. As has been mentioned previously in the discussion dealing with phonemic mastery, the child seems to master sounds according to the ease of modification of the breath stream, with the earliest consonants being those which require the least modification of the breath stream.

Nasal consonants involve a redirection of the breath stream through the nasal cavity, but the breath stream continues without interruption. The plosives require relatively uncomplicated modification of the breath stream, stopping of the stream momentarily and then releasing it again with a build up of breath pressure prior to release. Word lists for fricatives and affricates are the last groups of single consonants. Fricatives involve subtle modifications of the breath stream through narrowing and restricting the size of the oral channel. Affricates or combinations involve features of both plosives and fricatives.

The second and third dimensions, placement and voicing, provide more specific information concerning individual phonemes. For example, as will be seen from the descriptions which follow, when the breath stream is stopped for the plosives, the placement for the stop is either the lips, the tongue tip as it contacts the alveolar ridge or front of the hard palate, or the back of the tongue as it contacts the back of the soft palate.

Placement descriptions can never be exacting and precise because a specific sound may be produced correctly by a variety of different placements, depending on the oral structure and the phonetic context surrounding the consonant in question. Since the placement can vary so greatly, the so-called correct or acceptable placement for production of a particular phoneme during speech becomes an erroneous concept. The speech clinician who spends extensive time illustrating a specific placement for a specific sound commits a blunder. We all know of youngsters with severe malocclusions who manage to produce an acceptable /s/ through compensatory movement, and others with normal occlusion who distort this sound. There is no one placement for production of a sound, but there are placements, and the youngster finds his own placement in the process of phonemic maturation. This aspect will be developed further in a subsequent section. Composite word lists appear in this book grouping sounds similar in the placement dimension.

The voicing attribute refers to the absence of vocal cord vibrations, voiceless sounds, or the presence of vocal cord vibrations, voiced sounds. There are more voiced consonant sounds than voiceless. Templin found that these were among the last of the phoneme contrasts to be learned. Voicing errors have been found to be a chief error in the speech of early elementary school age children (Roe and Milisen, 1942). Voicing distinctions are particularly important with cleft palate patients who have difficulty developing sufficient intraoral breath pressure for production of voiceless consonants. Consonant function is also significant with cleft palate speakers, with better production, usually, for arresting consonants than for releasing consonants. The drill book contains lists made up of contrasting word pairs which differ only with respect to the voicing dimension. In order to have enough words, some words in the voicing contrast list are beyond the fourth grade reading level.

In summary, the over-all order of the word lists contained in the following pages utilizes multiple dimensions. The initial word lists emphasize sounds found to be mastered earliest by children, and later word lists emphasize sounds found to be mastered last by children. Each individual list is organized according to the function of the consonant phoneme as either that of releasing or arresting the breath stream. The number of syllables and phonemic elements contained by each word also receives consideration in the formation of the lists. Extended utterances involving phrases of two, three, and four words in length and all types of structurally complete sentences can be formed easily from the isolated word lists grouped according to parts of speech. Illustrations have been given of the many different phrases and sentences which can result from the lists. Final consideration is a phonetic classification of specific consonant phonemes according to manner, placement and voicing. There are word lists made up of contrasting word pairs differing only in the dimension of voicing, and also contrasting word lists grouped according to sounds which are similar in placement. These kinds of lists will facilitate results in therapy, as will be seen later.

The specific word lists follow in the order which has been described previously, according to the apparent ease of learning by the child and the complexity of the breath stream modification.

2. Drill Materials

CONSONANTS I

NASAL CONSONANTS

The three nasal consonants /m/, /n/, and /ŋ/ occur as the breath stream is directed through the nasal cavity, because passage through the mouth is closed completely at some point and the velum is open. The production of the three sounds differs only in the point at which the mouth passage is closed. For production of /m/, the mouth passage is closed because of the occlusion of the lips. For /n/ elevation of the tongue tip into contact with the palate or alveolar ridge closes the mouth passage, and for /ŋ/ nasal production occurs as the rear portion of the tongue contacts the velum. This latter sound functions as an arresting element only in the syllable and never functions as a releasing element. Word lists containing these sounds follow.

/m/, Arrest

First Syllable Arrest

Nouns		Verbs		Adjectives	Other
beam	limb	am	shame	dim	from
bomb	name	aim	blame	dumb	him
broom	room	came	scream	lame	them
charm	sum	come	storm	same	
dam	time	climb	bloom	some	
dime	cream	form	swim	simple	
farm	dream	frame	compare	clumsy	
game	drum	roam	compel	compact	
gem	flame	seem	complain	complete	
gum	frame		complete	ambitious	
ham	chimney		compose	important	
home	combat		embrace	comfortable	
lamb	comrade		employ	impossible	
lime	empire		gamble		
	family		impress		
	lumber				
	number				
	temper				
	ambition				

14

Nouns (cont.)

champion
companion
company
emperor
sympathy
combination
temperature

Second Syllable Arrest

Nouns	Verbs	Adjectives	Other
autumn	condemn	handsome	welcome
bathroom	inform		
bottom	exclaim		
column			

Third Syllable Arrest

Nouns	Verbs
uniform	overcome
telegram	

/m/, Release

First Syllable Release

Nouns			Verbs	Adjectives	Other
maid	month	morning	may	my	me
mail	mouth	mother	mow	mad	
man	machine	mountain	made	main	
map	mailbox	movie	make	mean	
match	manger	muscle	meet	more	
meat	marble	music	mess	much	
men	mansion	mustard	mile	mild	
mess	market	magazine	miss	most	
mice	mattress	manager	move	magic	
mill	meadow	medicine	march	many	
moon	measles	messenger	mark	maple	
mop	medal	microscope	melt	marble	
moth	message	minister	mend	merry	
mouse	minute	mosquito	mind	messy	
mouth	mirror	mystery	mix	metal	
mud	mitten	macaroni	must	million	
mule	money	motorcycle	marry	modern	
mask	monkey		murder	mischievous	
milk			multiply	magnificent	
			manufacture		

Second Syllable Release

Nouns	Verbs	Adjectives	Other
army	amuse	amazing	almost
chairman	amount	charming	among
damage	admire	common	tomorrow
farmer	admit	famous	
hammer	command	commercial	
humor	commence	familiar	
woman	commit	remarkable	
women	promise		
commission	remain		
committee	remark		
tomato	remind		
	remove		
	diminish		
	imitate		
	communicate		

Third Syllable Release

Nouns	Verbs
animal	recommend
apartment	
appointment	
equipment	
automobile	

Fourth Syllable Release

Nouns
advertisement
disappointment
experiment

/n/, Arrest

First Syllable Arrest

Nouns			Verbs		Adjectives	Other
barn	pen	throne	earn	sign	one	an
bean	pin	train	own	turn	fine	in
bone	rain	angel	burn	win	main	on
chain	scene	bandage	can	drown	mean	down
chin	sign	candy	dine	grin	pine	mine
cone	sin	concert	gain	plan	ten	soon
den	son	contest	lean	answer	thin	then
fun	sun	dentist	pain	conclude	worn	when
hen	thorn	donkey	phone	conquer	clean	instead
horn	town	general	ran	enjoy	green	into
line	wren	insect	run	insist	plain	only
man	yarn	insult	ruin	wander	plenty	lonely
men	brain	painter	seen	wonder	unhappy	under
moon	plane	pencil	shine	indicate		unless
pain	queen	princess				until
pan	skin	window				
	spoon	winter				
	stone					

Second Syllable Arrest

Nouns		Verbs	Adjectives	Other
iron	machine	open	broken	again
lion	mitten	began	divine	between
bargain	orphan	begin	eighteen	even
baron	poison	begun	million	upon
burden	prison	combine	seven	certainly
children	reason	define	sixteen	
chicken	season	fallen	sudden	
cotton	wagon	happen		
curtain	woman	listen		
cousin	women	remain		
engine	adventure	resign		
fortune	agency	complain		
garden	calendar			
kitten				

Third Syllable Arrest

Nouns	Verbs
champion	awaken
citizen	
companion	
decision	
physician	
telephone	

/n/, Release

First Syllable Release

Nouns		Verbs	Adjectives	Other
knee	note	know	new	no
knew	nurse	knock	neat	now
knot	nut	knit	nice	near
knife	noise	need	next	nor
knight	nest	nod	nasty	not
nail	navy	neglect	naughty	neither
nest	nectar	notice	narrow	never
news	needle		nervous	nothing
neck	neighbor		noble	
net	nephew			
niece	number			
night	newspaper			
north				
nose				

Second Syllable Release

Nouns		Verbs	Adjectives	Other
canoe	peanut	annoy	any	beneath
colonel	pony	banish	enough	anybody
dinner	senate	connect	honest	anyhow
harness	animal	deny	funny	anyone
manner	manager	finish	many	anything
money	phonograph	manage	tiny	anyway
morning	senator	punish	another	
penny	uniform		enormous	
planet				

Third Syllable Release

Nouns	Adjectives
criminal	definite
piano	

/ŋ/, Arrest

First Syllable Arrest

Nouns	Verbs	Adjectives
gang	hang	long
king	hung	wrong
ring	rang	young
song	sang	angry
thing	sing	hungry
wing	bring	single
swing		
spring		
string		
anger		
ankle		
finger		
hunger		
language		

Second and Third Syllable Arrest

Nouns	Adjectives	Other
building	surprising	along
evening		among
meeting		concerning
morning		
nothing		
something		

CONSONANTS II

PLOSIVES

The plosives are sounds resulting from a sudden stopping of the breath stream, impounding of pressure, and then release. This stopping, impounding, and release of the breath stream occurs at the precise points where passage through the mouth is closed for production of the nasal consonants. /m/ occurs as the lips seal off the oral passage, but the /p/ and /b/ occur as the breath stream is stopped and released through the mouth at the level of the lips. /n/ occurs as the action of the tongue tip and palate seal off the oral passage, but /t/ and /d/ occur as the breath stream is stopped and released through the mouth at this point. /ŋ/ occurs because the rear portion of the tongue and the palate seal off the oral passage, but /k/ and /g/ occur as the breath stream is stopped and released orally at this point. The voiced plosives are /b/, /d/, and /g/, and voice occurs at the moment of release of the consonants. The voiceless correlatives are /p/, /t/, and /k/, and there is a strong release of breath between the release of these consonants and beginning of voice for the following vowel. Word lists for each of these sounds follow. Contrasting lists of word pairs are presented differing only with respect to the voicing dimension.

/p/, Arrest

First Syllable Arrest

Nouns	Verbs	Adjectives	Other
ape	chop	cheap	up
cap	lap	deep	
cape	hop	ripe	
cup	hope	steep	
heap	keep		
lap	leap		
lip	ship		
map	tap		
mop	tip		
nap	whip		
rope	wipe		
shape	clap		
sheep	creep		
ship	drop		
soup	grip		
tape	sleep		
top			

Nouns (cont.)   *Verbs (cont.)*

whip	snap
crop	stoop
grip	stop
group	trap
step	capture
strip	upset
captain	
chapter	

Second Syllable Arrest

Nouns   *Verbs*

friendship	escape
equipment	

/p/, Release

First Syllable Release

Nouns		Verbs		Adjectives	Other
pea	painter	pay	push	pale	past
pie	palace	paid	put	pink	
paw	pencil	pain	patch	poor	
pack	penny	pass	pinch	pure	
page	pickle	pat	paint	painful	
pain	picture	pet	park	perfect	
path	pigeon	pick	paste	possible	
peach	pillow	pitch	point	peculiar	
pear	pilot	pour	polish		
pearl	picture	pull	punish		
pen	pocket				
pet	poem				
piece	police				
pig	pony				
pile	powder				
pin	puzzle				
pit	piano				
pole	potato				
pot					
purse					
paint					
park					
paste					
porch					

Second Syllable Release

Nouns		Verbs	Adjectives	Other
apple	opinion	appear	happy	upon
carpet	sympathy	appoint	rapid	
chapel	competition	compare	sleepy	
slipper	expedition	depart	stupid	
temper	experience	depend	apparent	
weapon	experiment	happen	capable	
appetite	operation	oppose	important	
capital	opinion	repay	opposite	
champion	opportunity	repeat	impossible	
company	superintendent	suppose		
department		deposit		
		operate		

Third Syllable Release

Nouns	Verbs	Adjectives
grasshopper	disappear	unhappy
caterpillar	disappoint	independent
independence	occupy	unexpected

/b/, Arrest

First Syllable Arrest

Noun	Verb
cube	rob
knob	rub
rib	sob
robe	grab
tub	
tube	
scab	
tribe	
subject	
submarine	
substitute	

Second Syllable Arrest

Verb
describe
disturb

/b/, Release

First Syllable Release

Nouns		Verbs	Adjectives	Other
bee	belt	be	bad	by
bow	bench	buy	bare	but
boy	best	bow	bald	barely
back	board	bake	best	because
bag	bond	bathe	bold	before
ball	box	beat	born	behind
bar	bulb	beg	better	behold
bath	bump	bite	busy	below
beach	balance	bet	beautiful	beneath
bear	banjo	bit		beside
bed	barrel	bid		between
beef	bargain	boil		beyond
beer	basement	bud		
bell	basket	bought		
bike	battle	burn		
bird	beggar	bark		
boat	bottle	bend		
bone	birthday	bent		
book	bucket	boast		
bowl	bugle	build		
bud	bullet	built		
bull	butcher	burst		
bun	butter	bust		
bus	button	become		
bush	business	became		
band	butterfly	began		
bank		begin		
barn		behave		
beard		believe		
		belong		
		betray		

Second Syllable Release

Nouns		Verbs	Adjectives
cabbage	robin	combine	able
combat	table	forbid	noble
hobby	timber	gamble	rubber
football	ambition	obey	ambitious
labor	nobody	tremble	forbidden
lumber	combination		
neighbor	laboratory		
number			
rabbit			

Contrasting Word Pairs Differing Only with the /p/ and /b/ Phonemes

/p/	/b/
pea	bee
pie	buy
pat	bat
pad	bad
pass	bass
path	bath
pan	ban
peg	beg
pet	bet
pen	Ben
pig	big
pail	bail
park	bark
pull	bull
pea	be
pear	bear
pour	bore
pin	bin
puff	buff
pest	best
pun	bun
pox	box
cap	cab
cup	cub
rip	rib
rope	robe
tap	tab
mop	mob

/t/, Arrest

First Syllable Arrest

Nouns			Verbs		Adjectives	Other
oat	heat	rate	ate	light	eight	it
boat	height	route	eat	meet	fat	at
boot	knot	vote	bit	might	hot	out
cat	light	sight	bite	write	date	but
coat	lot	weight	bought	pat	neat	not
date	meat	fleet	caught	pet	right	what
debt	net	flight	cut	put	wet	yet
dirt	night	fruit	doubt	set	white	quite
dot	note	scout	fight	sit	bright	lately
feet	nut	skate	fit	shot	flat	outside
foot	oat	football	get	shout	great	
gate	pet		hate	shut	sweet	
goat	pit		got	vote		
hat	pot		hit	wait		
	rat		let	float		
				greet		
				plate		
				split		

Second Syllable Arrest

Nouns		Verbs		Adjectives	Other
carpet	limit	admit	forget	complete	despite
closet	market	await	forgot	polite	except
debate	minute	commit	invite	private	completely
delight	pilot	defeat	repeat	quiet	
desert	planet	depart	salute	desperate	
diet	rabbit	devote	submit		
		dispute	visit		

Third Syllable Arrest

Nouns	Verbs	Adjectives
benefit	deposit	chocolate
cigarette		delicate
democrat		opposite

/t/, Release

First Syllable Release

Nouns		Verbs	Adjectives	Other
tie	table	tie	two	to
toe	teacher	take	tall	too
teeth	temper	talk	tame	today
time	temple	tap	ten	toward
tin	tunnel	teach	tin	together
tip	turkey	tear	tired	tomorrow
tire	tablespoon	tell	torn	
toad	telegram	took	tiny	
ton	telephone	toss	terrible	
tone	temperature	touch		
tooth		turn		
top		type		
tongue		told		
town		tumble		

Second Syllable Release

Nouns		Verbs	Adjectives		Other
actor	metal	attach	better	artificial	after
altar	motor	attack	bitter	particular	into
daughter	party	attend	guilty		until
hotel	plenty	contain	certain		certainly
autumn	safety	enter	dirty		entirely
beauty	sister	frighten	eighteen		yesterday
bottom	victim	intend	eighty		
butter	water	pity	empty		
city	writer	practice	entire		
center	article	return	fifteen		
curtain	attention	continue	fifty		
chapter	attorney	determine	forty		
cotton	interview	interview	fourteen		
county	photograph		mighty		
critic	victory		pretty		
doctor	intelligence		sixty		
letter	material		sixteen		
matter			beautiful		

/t/, Release

Third Syllable Release

Nouns	Adjectives
committee	uncertain
liberty	
quality	
senator	
visitor	
competition	
invitation	
military	

Fourth-Fifth Syllable Release

Nouns
majority
personality

/d/, Arrest

First Syllable Arrest

Nouns	Verbs	Adjectives
bead	add	bad
bed	feed	sad
bird	had	good
food	heard	mad
head	hide	red
load	lead	wide
mud	load	glad
road	made	
seed	paid	
shade	read	
sword	ride	
weed	rode	
wood	said	
bread		
cloud		
sled		
spade		
thread		

Second Syllable Arrest

Nouns	Adjectives
parade	absurd

/d/, Release

First Syllable Release

Nouns		Verbs		Adjectives	Other
day	dish	die	dig	deaf	down
dew	dog	do	dine	dear	
dance	door	dance	dip	deep	
deck	duck	dare	does	dim	
deer	desk	deal	declare	dark	
dime	daisy	dial	discuss	damp	
	danger			dirty	
	diary			delicious	
				dangerous	

Second and Third Syllable Release

Nouns		Verbs	Adjectives	Other
candy	soda	wonder	muddy	under
garden	spider		ready	today
ladder	window		shady	
lady	wedding		medical	
meadow	Indian			
radish	medicine			
reindeer	radio			
shadow	nobody			
	somebody			

Contrasting Word Pairs Differing Only with the /t/ and /d/ Phonemes

/t/	/d/
to	do
toe	dough
tall	doll
tie	die
ten	den
town	down
tear	dear
tear	dare
tore	door
tuck	duck
ton	done
hit	hid
at	add
cat	cad
cut	cud
coat	code
cot	cod
not	nod
late	laid
hat	had
bat	bad
bet	bed
mut	mud
mate	made
ant	and
colt	cold
try	dry

/k/, Arrest

First Syllable Arrest

Nouns		Verbs		Adjectives	Other
back	block	ache	seek	oak	back
book	brake	bark	shake	sick	likely
check	flake	fake	shock	dark	
cheek	flock	check	shook	black	
deck	smoke	choke	soak	successful	
dock	snake	lack	talk		
duck	steak	leak	take		
hook	truck	lick	took		
hawk	stick	like	walk		
lake	strike	lock	blink		
luck	backbone	look	break		
neck	blackboard	make	broke		
rock	breakfast	pack	smoke		
sock	picture	peck	sneak		
bark	accident	pick	speak		
		rake	spoke		
			strike		
			accept		
			succeed		

Second and Third Syllable Arrest

Nouns	Verbs	Adjectives
attack	attack	magic
mistake	overlook	electric
affection		

/k/, Release

First Syllable Release

Nouns		Verbs		Adjectives
key	card	call	count	cool
cab	cart	came	cost	cold
cage	court	can	carry	kind
can	canal	care	complete	calm
cap	canoe	catch	confess	careful
car	candy	caught	connect	copper
cat	captain	comb	copy	correct
cave	carpet	come	correct	curious
coat	carriage	cut		cunning
coin	castle	keep		comfortable
comb	country	kill		
cot	courage	kiss		
cup	cousin	carve		
cough	color			
curb	collar			
curse	contest			
king	kitchen			
kite	carpenter			
camp	company			
	caterpillar			

Second Syllable Release

Nouns		Verbs	Adjectives	Other
acre	second	occur	local	because
chicken	turkey	record	lucky	welcome
circle	stocking	decorate	naked	according
market	ticket	occupy	second	
pocket	handkerchief	recognize	wicked	
record		recommend		
		recover		

Third and Fourth Syllable Release

Nouns	Verbs	Adjectives
article	educate	medical
application	overcome	physical
	electrocute	practical
		particular

/g/, Arrest

First Syllable Arrest

Nouns	Verbs	Adjectives
egg	beg	big
bag	dig	vague
bug	dug	ignorant
dog	hug	magnificent
fig	tag	
fog	tug	
jug	wag	
hog	drag	
leg		
league		
log		
pig		
rag		
rug		
wig		
drug		
flag		
frog		

/g/, Release

First Syllable Release

Nouns		Verbs	Adjectives	Other
gain	gun	go	gay	gone
game	gift	gave	good	
gate	guest	gaze	gold	
geese	garden	get	gallant	
goat	governor	give	guilty	
goose	government	got	golden	
girl		goes		
gum		guess		
		guide		
		guard		

Second and Third Syllable Release

Nouns	Verbs	Adjectives	Other
bargain	argue	eager	ago
eagle	began	legal	again
organ	begin	regular	regard
sugar	forget		together
tiger	forgive		altogether
wagon	forgot		
agony	stagger		
argument	organize		
magazine			

Contrasting Word Pairs Differing Only with the /g/ and /k/ Phonemes

/g/	/k/
game	came
goat	coat
girl	curl
gum	come
gave	cave
got	cot
guard	card
good	could
gold	cold
bag	back
bug	buck
dig	Dick
dug	duck
lug	luck
pig	pick
rag	rack
tag	tack
tug	tuck
wig	wick
peg	peck
glass	class
grow	crow
grew	crew
great	crate
ground	crowned

CONSONANTS III

SEMIVOWELS

Semivowels resemble vowels, but there is some slight interference to the breath stream and the oral channel is more constricted than in most vowels. Following Templin's classification, the glides /w/ and /j/ as well as /h/ and /l/ will be treated as semivowels. The /r/ is not treated as a semivowel here but will be handled separately with accompanying word lists. The breath stream is not the significant feature with the semivowels, as has been noted with the nasals and plosives, and as will be noted with the fricatives.

The glides /j/ and /w/ are characterized by movement toward the sound which follows. Each glide is characterized by movement in a particular direction and not movement to one definite position. Separate lists are not made here for the /hw/ because so few persons make a distinction between /w/ and /hw/. Fairbanks (1960) mentions that fewer people actually use the latter sound and Templin found this to be true also with most of her children (1957). Words containing /wh/, however, are separated from the /w/ words for those who produce this sound. The articulatory position for /h/ also becomes that of the vowel sound which follows and is similar to a whispering of that vowel. This sound functions to release the syllable pulse only. The glides /w/ and /j/ also release the syllable pulse only.

The final sound included among the semivowels is /l/, which is produced when the tongue tip is elevated to loosely contact the alveolar ridge or hard palate, with the breath stream passing around the loose edges of the tongue. It will be remembered that, if firm contact of the tongue tip is maintained against the hard palate, the nasal consonant /n/ is produced, but if release is made from the tight contact the plosives /t/ and /d/ will result. The [l] arresting the breath stream may function as a semivowel in the words *bell* and *ball* or it may function as a vowel in the words *buckle* and *wrinkle*. Lists follow, with a separate list for [l] as a semivowel and for [l] as a vowel.

/h/, Release

First Syllable Release

Nouns		Verbs	Adjectives	Other
hay	hand	had	high	her
hail	harp	hail	hot	who
hair	haste	has	whole	hardly
hat	health	hate	whose	hello
hate	heart	haul	happy	highly
hawk	herd	have	heavy	himself
head	habit	heal	helpless	herself
heat	hammer	hear	holy	heavily
hedge	handle	heard	hundred	
heel	harbor	heed	horrible	
height	harness	hide		
hen	harvest	hop		
hill	heaven	hurt		
home	helmet	held		
horse	hero	harm		
house	highway	haunt		
	honey	hold		
	hotel	hunt		
	humor	happen		
	hunter	hurry		
	husband	hesitate		

Second Syllable Release

Nouns	Verbs	Other
grasshopper	behave	behind
schoolhouse	beheld	behold
		perhaps
		somehow

/j/, Release

First Syllable Release

Nouns	Verbs	Adjectives	Other
year	yell	your	you
youth		young	yes
yard		yellow	yet
yesterday		youthful	yours
			yonder

Second and Third Syllable Release

Nouns	Verbs	Adjectives	Other
lawyer	argue	brilliant	beyond
mayor		junior	
onion		loyal	
union		million	
argument		familiar	
companion		peculiar	
opinion			

/w/, Release

First Syllable Release

Nouns		Verbs		Adjectives	Other
way	worm	weigh	worry	weak	we
walk	wound	wail	worship	wet	well
wake	wagon	wait		wide	with
wall	water	wake	*wh*	wise	widely
war	weapon	walk	whip	worse	within
wash	weather	was	whisper	warm	without
watch	wedding	wash	whistle	wild	
wax	widow	watch		worn	*wh*
weed	willow	wave		worst	why
weak	window	wear		wealthy	what
weight	winter	weave		weary	when
wife	wisdom	weep		western	where
wine	witness	were		wicked	which
wish	woman	will		wonderful	while
witch	women	win			whether
wood	worker	wipe		*wh*	
wool	warrior	wish		white	
word	wilderness	won			
work		worth			
waist	*wh*	would			
west	wheat	want			
width	wheel	waste			
wolf	whip	went			
world		wept			
		wink			

Second and Third Syllable Release

Nouns	Verbs	Adjectives	Other
doorway	await	awake	away
highway	forward	aware	always
language	reward	backward	farewell
reward			anyone
sandwich			anyway
			everyone
			wh
			anywhere

Semivowel [l], Arrest

First Syllable Arrest

Nouns		Verbs		Adjectives	Other
oil	pearl	boil	tell	ill	well
ball	pill	call	toil	pale	while
bell	pile	chill	will	pearl	also
coal	pole	curl	yell	real	always
doll	pool	fail	spill	tall	
fuel	sail	fall	steal	still	
girl	shell	feel	stole	swell	
hall	sole	fill		steel	
heel	school	haul		healthy	
hill	wall	heal		selfish	
hole	wheel	howl		welcome	
fail	yell	kill			
mail	steel	pile			
male	trail	pull			
meal	railroad	sail			
mile	soldier	sell			
mill					
mule					
nail					

Second, Third, and Fourth Syllable Arrest

Nouns	Verbs	Adjectives	Other
hotel	quarrel	vital	until
squirrel		peaceful	
automobile		beautiful	
		natural	
		powerful	

Semivowel [l], Release

First Syllable Release

Nouns	Verbs	Adjectives
law	lay	low
lace	lie	lame
lad	lack	late
lake	lace	lean
lamb	laid	less
lap	lash	lone
lawn	laugh	long
league	lead	loose
leg	leap	large
life	led	last
light	leave	left
lip	let	latter
loan	lick	lazy
lock	light	little
log	like	lower
luck	live	lucky
lamp	learn	
land	lock	
list	look	
lunch	lose	
lady	love	
laughter	lend	
lawyer	lift	
leader	lost	
lecture	listen	
lemon	locate	
lesson		
liquid		
library		

Second Syllable Release

Nouns	Verbs	Adjectives	Other
belief	allow	holy	alike
ceiling	believe	jealous	below
challenge	belong	polite	hardly
college	collect	delicate	hello
color	delay	eleven	only
dollar	delight	foolish	really
family	elect	solid	sadly
pillow	follow	useless	truly
police	gallop	yellow	unless
policeman	polish		
elephant	release		
religion	salute		
ruler			
sailor			
telephone			
telegram			

Third and Fourth Syllable Release

Nouns	Verbs	Adjectives	Other
ability	realize	chocolate	certainly
envelope		excellent	exactly
violet		popular	honestly
population			perfectly
			recently
			especially

Vocalic [l]

Nouns		Verbs	Adjectives
angle	tunnel	marvel	pale
ankle	uncle	travel	ample
apple	article	tumble	final
battle			metal
bubble			noble
candle			purple
chapel			simple
circle			medical
couple			physical
devil			remarkable
kettle			
marble			
metal			
muscle			
pencil			
people			
puzzle			
rattle			
saddle			
sparkle			
table			
title			
criminal			

CONSONANTS IV

FRICATIVES

The fricatives occur as the breath stream passing through a restricted channel contacts the teeth, tongue, lips, alveolar ridge, or hard palate. A friction-like noise occurs as the breath stream passes over one or more than one of the articulators. Fricatives are continuants requiring continuous egress of the breath stream and not a stopping of the breath stream as with plosives. Relatively fine tongue control is required for correct production of all of the fricatives. The fricatives are /f/ and /v/; /ə/ and /ð/; /s/ and /z/; /ʃ/ and /ʒ/. The first of each of the paired sounds is voiceless, and the second is voiced.

Individual fricatives differ by virtue of the size and shape of the opening through which the breath stream passes. The so-called slit fricatives are produced with an opening which is relatively wide from side to side and narrow from top to bottom; grooved fricatives are narrower from side to side and deeper from top to bottom. The first four fricatives (/f/, /v/, /ə/, and /ð/) are slit fricatives and the last four (/s/, /z/, /ʃ/, and /ʒ/) are grooved fricatives (Gleason, 1955, pages 22-23). Word lists for each of the fricatives follow. Contrasting lists of word pairs are presented differing only with respect to the dimension of voicing.

/f/, Arrest

First Syllable Arrest

Nouns	Verbs	Adjectives	Other
chief	laugh	brief	if
hoof		rough	off
knife		safe	safely
leaf		difficult	
life			
puff			
roof			
thief			
wife			
grief			
staff			
stuff			
difference			
laughter			
safety			
afternoon			

Second and Third Syllable Arrest

Nouns
belief
mischief
relief
sheriff
handkerchief
telegraph

/f/, Release

First Syllable Release

Nouns		Verbs	Adjectives	Other
fee	favor	fade	four	far
face	feather	fail	fair	for
fun	fellow	fall	fat	forth
fan	female	fed	few	fairly
fire	fever	feed	full	farther
fish	finger	feel	fine	farewell
faith	football	fell	fast	finally
fear	forest	fetch	first	forever
feet	fortune	fill	fond	formerly
fence	future	fish	fierce	
food	physician	fit	famous	
fool		fix	fancy	
foot		felt	final	
force		find	foolish	
file		fold	foreign	
phone		found	formal	
fact		finish	former	
farm		follow	forty	
fault		forget	familiar	
field		forgot	favorite	
force		furnish	forgotten	
fort			fortunate	
fairy			favorable	
farmer				
fashion				
father				

Second Syllable Release

Nouns	Verbs	Adjectives	Other
affair	afford	careful	before
breakfast	confess	dreadful	definitely
coffee	defeat	peaceful	
comfort	defend	selfish	
defense	differ	youthful	
effect	inform	definite	
effort	offend	sufficient	
office	offer	comfortable	
profit	perform	unfortunate	
rifle	prefer		
surface	suffer		
traffic			
affection			
officer			
performance			
professor			
information			

Third and Fourth Syllable Release

Nouns	Verbs	Adjectives
benefit	justify	artificial
elephant	satisfy	beautiful
telephone	identify	powerful
satisfaction		successful
		wonderful
		scientific

/v/, Arrest

First Syllable Arrest

Nouns	Verbs	Adjectives	Other
cave	carve	brave	of
nerve	dive	every	lovely
glove	gave	several	everybody
grave	give	evident	everyone
slave	have		
sleeve	leave		
stove	live		
movement	love		
	move		
	save		
	wave		
	weave		
	drive		
	drove		
	prove		

Second, Third, and Fourth Syllable Arrest

Nouns	Verbs	Adjectives	Other
motive	achieve	native	above
discovery	approve	primitive	
achievement	believe		
executive	conceive		
	deceive		
	derive		
	dissolve		
	forgive		
	observe		
	receive		
	relieve		
	remove		
	reserve		
	resolve		

/v/, Release

First Syllable Release

Nouns	Verbs	Adjectives	Other
view	vow	vain	very
van	vote	vague	even
veil	vanish	vast	over
vein	visit	vital	
vine		violent	
verse		visible	
voice		valuable	
vote		various	
valley			
value			
vessel			
victim			
village			
virtue			
vision			
volume			
voyage			
vacation			
violence			
violet			
visitor			
vegetable			

Second and Third Syllable Release

Nouns		Verbs	Adjectives	Other
advice	envelope	cover	divine	moreover
device	governor	advance	heavy	
devil	invention	advise	nervous	
divorce	conversation	avoid	private	
driver	development	convert	seven	
heaven	invitation	convince	severe	
movie	civilization	divide	silver	
navy	investigation	devote	convenient	
oven	interval	envy	obvious	
river	observer	invest	previous	
advantage		invent	seventy	
adventure		provide	seventeen	
		prevail	eleven	
		prevent		
		revenge		
		reveal		
		develop		
		cultivate		
		deliver		
		discover		
		interview		

Contrasting Word Pairs Differing Only with the /f/ and /v/ Phonemes

/f/	/v/
few	view
fine	vine
fan	van
fat	vat
file	vile
fault	vault
feel	veal
fast	vast
fail	veil
ferry	very
half	have
safe	save
leaf	leave
proof	prove
belief	believe
relief	relieve

/θ/, Arrest

First Syllable Arrest

Nouns	Verbs	Adjectives	Other
earth	withdraw	fourth	with
bath		fifth	
birth		worth	
breath		ninth	
cloth		faithful	
death		youthful	
faith			
health			
month			
mouth			
north			
path			
south			
strength			
teeth			
tooth			
truth			
wealth			
youth			
birthday			

/θ/, Release

First Syllable Release

Nouns	Verbs	Adjectives
thief	thank	thigh
thing	thought	thin
thorn		third
thirst		thirsty
theater		thirty
thunder		thirteen
		thousand

Second and Third Syllable Release

Nouns	Adjectives	Other
nothing	healthy	within
something	wealthy	without
authority		
sympathy		

/ð/, Arrest

First Syllable Arrest

Nouns	Verbs	Adjectives
bathe	breathe	smooth
	clothe	

/ð/, Release

First Syllable Release

		Adjectives	Other
		this	the
		these	them
		that	there
		those	than
		their	they

Second and Third Syllable Release

Nouns	Verbs	Adjectives	Other
brother	bother	other	either
clothing	gather	leather	farther
father		worthy	further
feather			neither
leather			together
mother			
grandfather			
grandmother			

/s/, Arrest

First Syllable Arrest

Nouns		Verbs	Adjectives	Other
ice	dance	chase	lace	us
base	peace	cross	loose	else
boss	rice	curse	nice	once
bus	cross	dance	this	yes
case	dress	guess	brass	closely
chance	grass	kiss	fierce	elsewhere
gas	history	lace	distant	especially
goose	yesterday	miss	useful	
horse		pass		
house		bless		
mice		dress		
mouse		discharge		
class		dislike		
		whisper		

Second Syllable Arrest

Nouns	Verbs	Adjectives	Other
congress	confess	careless	across
canvas	convince	cautious	
darkness	decrease	conscious	
device	divorce	famous	
difference	embrace	helpless	
divorce		jealous	
witness		nervous	
policeman		domestic	

Third Syllable Arrest

Nouns	Adjectives
evidence	curious
	dangerous
	delicious
	previous
	glorious
	religious

/s/, Release

First Syllable Release

Nouns		Verbs		Adjectives	Other
sea	sandwich	saw	sit	sad	so
sack	savage	see	soak	safe	soon
sauce	season	say	send	same	sadly
seat	secret	sew	sent	sick	safely
seed	salary	said	sink	seven	seldom
side	senator	sail	salute	soft	simply
sign	summer	sang	select	some	softly
soap	sunshine	sank	soften	sore	somehow
soil		sat	submit	such	sometime
son		save	suffer	severe	silently
song		search	celebrate	silly	suddenly
soup		seek	satisfy	simple	sufficiently
suit		seem	separate	single	
salt		seen		sober	
sand		seize		solemn	
silk		sell		solid	
ceiling		serve		sorry	
saddle		set		sudden	
sailor		sing		sunny	

Second, Third, and Fourth Syllable Release

Nouns	Verbs		Adjectives	Other
acid	absorb	whistle	absent	also
basin	accept	assemble	fancy	beside
blessing	answer	astonish	handsome	herself
concert	ascend	consider	recent	himself
consent	assault		absolute	inside
council	assign		possible	outside
lesson	conceal		uncertain	concerning
insect	concern		impossible	recently
pencil	consent		innocent	absolutely
person	consult		magnificent	
bicycle	consume			
decision	deceive			
comparison	decide			
conversation	descend			
professor	listen			
curiosity	pursue			
democracy	receive			
university	upset			

/z/, Arrest

First Syllable Arrest

Nouns	Verbs	Adjectives	Other
ease	is	his	as
cause	use	those	
cheese	chose	these	
rose	choose	wise	
breeze	close	whose	
clothes	does	wise	
husband	has		
	lose		
	raise		
	rise		
	was		

Second and Third Syllable Arrest

Verbs	Other
accuse	always
advise	because
amaze	afterwards
amuse	
arise	
arose	
arouse	
compose	
confuse	

/z/, Release

First and Second Syllable Release

Nouns	Verbs	Adjectives
zone	deserve	busy
closet	design	crazy
cousin	desire	easy
daisy	observe	frozen
dozen	reserve	lazy
music	resign	pleasant
peasant	visit	present
present		thousand
prison		musical
puzzle		physical
observe		desirable
reason		reasonable
resort		
result		
visitor		
physician		
position		
president		

Third and Fourth Syllable Release

Nouns	Verbs	Adjectives
magazine	deposit	opposite
advertising	represent	
organization		

Contrasting Word Pairs Differing Only
with the /s/ and /z/ Phonemes

/z/	/s/
zip	sip
zoo	sue
zeal	seal
zinc	sink
buzz	bus
plays	place
lose	loose
lies	lice
rise	rice
eyes	ice
his	hiss
use (v.)	use (n.)
fuzz	fuss
clothes	close (adj.)
raise	race
phase	face

/ʃ/, Arrest

First Syllable Arrest

Nouns	Verbs	Adjectives
ash	dash	fresh
bush	fish	
dish	push	
fish	rush	
brush	wash	
flash	wish	
splash	brush	
	crush	
	splash	

Second and Third Syllable Arrest

Nouns	Verbs	Adjectives
establishment	finish	foolish
	flourish	selfish
	perish	
	publish	
	vanish	
	establish	
	distinguish	

/ʃ/, Release

First Syllable Release

Nouns		Verbs		Adjectives	Other
shoe	shop	show	shut	shown	she
shade	shore	shake	should	short	sharply
shame	shield	shall	shiver	sharp	shortly
shape	shadow	share		shallow	
sheep	shelter	shine			
sheet	shepherd	shone			
shell	sheriff	shook			
ship	shoulder	shoot			
shirt	shower	shot			
shock	sugar	shout			

Second Syllable Release

Nouns		Verbs	Adjectives
action	pressure	worship	ashamed
bushel	portion		gracious
cushion	station		patient
machine	sunshine		precious
nation			social
ocean			special
patience			national

Third and Fourth Syllable Release

Nouns		Verbs	Adjectives	Other
addition	proportion	appreciate	delicious	especially
ambition	protection		commercial	sufficiently
attention	reaction		sufficient	
direction	reduction		professional	
election	reflection		presidential	
exception	sensation			
expression	suspicion			
foundation	vacation			
impression	admiration			
objection	expedition			
physician	explanation			
permission	illustration			
procession	introduction			
production	invitation			
profession	resolution			
	revolution			
	satisfaction			
	transportation			

/ʒ/, Release

Second Syllable Release

Nouns	Adjectives	Other
measure	usual	usually
vision		
pleasure		
treasure		
treasury		

Third Syllable Release

Nouns	Adjectives
conclusion	unusual
confusion	
decision	
division	
occasion	

CONSONANTS V

AFFRICATES OR COMBINATIONS (PLOSIVE AND FRICATIVE)

These sounds are referred to as combinations because their production involves the features of both the plosive (stopping and release of the breath stream) and the fricative (passing of the breath stream through a restricted channel or fricative position). Two sounds are involved, /tʃ/ and /dʒ/, the former voiceless and the latter voiced. Combination lists follow. Contrasting lists of word pairs will be presented differing only with respect to these two sound combinations.

/dʒ/, Arrest

First, Second, and Third Syllable Arrest

Nouns	Verbs	Adjectives	Other
age	urge	huge	strangely
cage	change	large	
edge	charge	strange	
page	arrange		
bridge	engage		
average	manage		
carriage	oblige		
college			
cottage			
courage			
language			
message			
orange			
package			
village			
arrangement			
advantage			

/dʒ/, Release

First Syllable Release

Nouns		Verbs	Adjectives	Other
joy	junior	join	just	gently
gem	jury	jump	gentle	just
jail	justice	justify	jealous	
jar	general		jolly	
job	gentleman			
joke	January			
juice				
joint				
June				
giant				
jacket				
Japan				
July				
jewel				
journal				
journey				

Second and Third Syllable Release

Nouns	Verbs	Adjectives
agent	digest	magic
angel	injure	major
danger	object	dangerous
pigeon	rejoice	original
soldier	suggest	
stranger		
agency		
engineer		
injury		
majority		
vegetable		
messenger		
origin		

/tʃ/, Arrest

First and Second Syllable Arrest

Nouns	Verbs	Adjectives	Other
each	catch	each	which
itch	march	much	
coach	match	rich	
couch	pitch	such	
lunch	reach	French	
march	search		
match	teach		
porch	touch		
ranch	watch		
watch	preach		
witch	snatch		
branch	attach		
speech	approach		
sandwich			

/tʃ/, Release

First Syllable Release

Nouns		Verbs	Adjectives	Other
chain	chin	change	cheap	chiefly
chair	child	chase	charming	
chance	chart	check	cheerful	
charm	chamber	cheer	chocolate	
check	channel	choke		
cheek	chapel	chop		
cheese	chapter	choose		
chief	cherry	challenge		
chill	chicken	chatter		
	children			
	chimney			
	champion			
	charity			

Second, Third, and Fourth Syllable Release

Nouns		Verbs	Adjectives	Other
butcher	structure	achieve	wretched	actually
discharge	century	discharge	actual	
kitchen	achievement	exchange	fortunate	
lecture	adventure	venture		
luncheon	handkerchief	manufacture		
mischief	agriculture			
picture	manufacturer			
pitcher				
teacher				

Contrasting Word Pairs Differing Only
with /tʃ/ and /dʒ/ Phonemes

/tʃ/	/dʒ/
chin	gin
chain	Jane
cherry	Jerry
cheer	jeer
choke	joke
cheap	jeep
etch	edge
match	Madge
march	Marge
lunch	lunge
rich	ridge
search	serge

CONSONANTS VI

/r/ SOUNDS

Four different /r/ sounds have recently been described (Curtis and Hardy, 1959). For reasons to be discussed later, drill material which follows will be presented for three /r/ sounds only, the consonant glide [r], the stressed vocalic [ɝ], and the unstressed vocalic [ɚ]. The /r/ at the ends of words will always be considered to be vocalic, either stressed or unstressed, thus not agreeing always with Kenyon and Knott (1944). In such words as *car* and *bear* the phoneme will be considered as an unstressed vocalic, since a substitution error for this sound is usually a vowel. The /r/ occurring in words such as *heart, card,* and *fork* will likewise be considered as unstressed vocalic—taking exception to Fairbanks' treatment (Fairbanks, 1960)—because of evidence from Curtis and Hardy, and because the sound functions more as a vowel than a consonant in these words. The vocalic [r]'s will be classified, according to the position in the word, as initial, medial, or final. When the sound is medial, the syllable in which it occurs will be specified.

The consonant glide [r] will be noted in such words as *row* and *story,* where it releases the syllable. The intervocalic [r] of Curtis and Hardy in such words as *carrot* and *arrow* will be classified here as a consonant glide, agreeing in this instance with Kenyon and Knott, because it is felt that for speaking purposes the /r/ releases the second syllable in the words. Errors involving the intervocalic [r] so-called are usually either omissions or substitutions involving another glide /w/ or /j/. In articulation training, results can be quicker if the child views the /r/ in these words as a consonant to release the second syllable, as a later section will describe.

Consonant Glide [r], Release

First Syllable Release

Nouns		Verbs		Adjectives	Other
ray	rush	race	relieve	raw	really
race	wreck	raise	remain	real	
rack	rabbit	ran	remind	red	
rag	rattle	reach	remove	rich	
rail	reason	read	renew	rid	
rain	receipt	reign	repeat	right	
ranch	region	ride	reply	ripe	
rank	relief	rise	replace	rough	
rat	rifle	rob	rescue	round	
ring	robber	rode	reveal	rude	
rent	robin	roll	review	rapid	
rib	wrinkle	rub	revolt	ready	
rice	radio	run	realize	recent	
ride	regiment	rush	recommend	reckless	
ridge	religion	wrap		remote	
road		wreck		royal	
robe		write		restless	
rock		wrote		wrong	
roof		risk		wretched	
room		receive		reasonable	
root		reckon		romantic	
rose		refuse		responsible	
rule		relate			

Second, Third, and Fourth Syllable Release

Nouns	Verbs	Adjectives	Other
arrow	arise	erect	around
barrel	arose	different	every
bedroom	arrange	favorite	very
berry	arrest	narrow	already
carrot	erect	sorry	directly
cherry	direct	generous	tomorrow
comrade		glorious	
fury		terrible	
glory		elaborate	
orange			
sorrow			
squirrel			
story			
arena			
direction			
variety			
cigarette			
luxury			
memory			
editorial			

Stressed Vocalic [ɝ]

Initial Position

Nouns	Verbs	Adjectives	Other
earth	earn	earnest	early
	urge		

Medial Position

First Syllable

Nouns	*Verbs*	*Adjectives*	*Other*
bird	burn	firm	firmly
church	curse	first	perfectly
curl	heard	worth	
curve	hurl	certain	
curse	hurt	dirty	
girl	learn	nervous	
nerve	turn	perfect	
nurse	work	thirty	
pearl	furnish	thirteen	
shirt		worthy	
spur		permanent	
worm		personal	
clerk			
birthday			
circle			
curtain			
journey			
permit			
person			
purpose			
turkey			
turtle			

Second Syllable

Nouns	*Verbs*	*Adjectives*	*Other*
desert	disturb	absurd	concerning
	observe	concerned	
		uncertain	

Final Position

Nouns	*Adjectives*
fir	fir
	her

Unstressed Vocalic [ɚ]

Medial Position

First Syllable

Nouns	Verbs	Adjectives	Other
arm	march	torn	sharply
barn	permit	marble	shortly
board	persuade	charming	
cart	start		
charm			
heart			
part			
sword			
bargain			
chairman			
morning			
orphan			

Second and Third Syllable

Nouns	Verbs	Adjectives	Other
blackboard	inform	modern	underneath
afternoon	overcome	important	yesterday
uniform		comfortable	

Final Position

First Syllable

Nouns	Verbs	Adjectives	Other
air	hear	clear	or
bear	pour	fair	near
bar	tear	four	where
car	tore	more	
chair	wear	sure	
deer	wore	your	
door			
ear			
fire			
hair			
star			
store			

Second Syllable

Nouns		Verbs	Adjectives	Other
affair	paper	answer	bitter	after
anchor	pepper	capture	clever	before
butter	pitcher	chatter	eager	either
center	powder	compare	inner	neither
chamber	sailor	desire	silver	over
chapter	soldier	enter	tender	under
danger	slipper	offer		
dinner	teacher	shiver		
father	temper	suffer		
flower	water	utter		
hammer	weather			
leader				
letter				
liquor				
master				
motor				
mother				
neighbor				
number				
odor				
owner				
painter				

Third Syllable

Nouns	Verbs	Adjectives	Other
adventure	deliver	another	anywhere
manager	discover		together
messenger			
passenger			

BLENDS I

/l/, /r/, AND /s/ BLENDS

While more than 150 consonant blends occur in the English language, many appear infrequently. The principal blends involve the /l/, /r/, and /s/ phonemes. Drill words containing two-element blends involving these three phonemes follow, in that order. Only three blends, /sk/, /sp/, and /st/, arrest and release the syllable; the other blends release the syllable only. Even /sk/ and /sp/ function relatively rarely to arrest the syllable.

TWO-ELEMENT BLENDS

[l] Blends

/bl/, Release

First and Second Syllable Release

Nouns	Verbs	Adjectives
black	blow	blue
blade	blew	black
blame	blame	blank
blank	blast	blind
blast	blaze	bloody
blaze	bless	
block	block	
blood	bloom	
blush	blush	
blessing	oblige	
blossom		

/fl/, Release

First Syllable Release

Nouns	Verbs	Adjectives
flag	flag	flat
flame	flame	
flash	flash	
flat	fled	
fleet	flew	
flesh	float	
flight	flood	
flock	flow	
flood	flung	
floor	flush	
flour	fly	
flush	flatter	
fly	flavor	
flavor	flourish	
flower	flower	
	flutter	

Second and Third Syllable Release

Nouns

conflict
influence
butterfly

/gl/, Release

First and Second Syllable Release

Nouns	Verbs	Adjectives
glance	glance	glad
glare	glare	glorious
glass	gleam	
gleam	glide	
glimpse	glimpse	
glove	glitter	
glitter	neglect	
glory		

/kl/, Release

First Syllable Release

Nouns		Verbs		Adjectives	Other
claw	cloth	claw	clothe	clean	clearly
clay	clothes	clad	clutch	clear	closely
claim	cloud	claim	cluster	close	
clasp	club	clap		clever	
class	clutch	clasp			
clerk	climate	class			
cliff	closet	clean			
climb	clothing	clear			
cloak	cluster	climb			
clock		cling			
close		close			

Second Syllable Release

Nouns	Verbs
incline	conclude
conclusion	declare
	include
	proclaim

/pl/, Release

First Syllable Release

Nouns	Verbs	Adjectives	Other
play	play	plain	please
place	plow	pleasant	plainly
plan	place	plenty	
plane	plan		
plant	plane		
plate	plant		
pledge	plead		
plot	please		
plow	pluck		
plum	plunge		
planet			
platform			
player			
pleasure			

Second Syllable Release

Nouns	Verbs	Adjectives	Other
display	apply	complete	completely
employer	complain		
employment	display		
	employ		
	explain		
	reply		
	replace		
	supply		

/sl/, Release

First and Second Syllable Release

Nouns	Verbs	Adjectives	Other
sleep	slay	slight	slightly
sleeve	slain	slow	slowly
slice	sleep	slender	asleep
slide	slept		
slip	slice		
slope	slide		
slavery	slip		
slipper	slow		
slowness	dislike		
slumber			

[r] Blends

/br/, Release

First Syllable Release

Nouns	Verbs	Adjectives	Other
brow	break	brief	briefly
brain	brush	bright	
brake	bring	broad	
branch	broke	brown	
brand	brought	brilliant	
brass		broken	
brave			
bread			
break			
breast			
breath			
breeze			
brick			
bride			
bridge			
brook			
brush			
brother			
breakfast			

Second Syllable Release

Nouns	Verbs	Adjectives	Other
fabric	embrace	celebrated	abroad
library	celebrate		
celebration			

/dr/, Release

First Syllable Release

Nouns	Verbs	Adjectives
dream	dry	dry
dress	draft	dreadful
drink	drain	dramatic
drop	drank	
drug	draw	
drum	dread	
drunk	dried	
dragon	drift	
drama	drill	
drawer	drive	
children	droop	
driver	drove	
	drown	

Second and Third Syllable Release

Nouns	Verbs	Adjectives
children	withdraw	hundred
cathedral		

/fr/, Release

First and Second Syllable Release

Nouns	Verbs	Adjectives	Other
frame	free	frank	from
freight	freeze	frequent	frankly
friend	fret	fresh	freely
fright	frown	friendly	frequently
frock	frighten	frozen	
frog		afraid	
front			
frost			
fruit			
phrase			
fragment			
freedom			
friar			
friendship			
frontier			

/gr/, Release

First Syllable Release

Nouns	Verbs	Adjectives	Other
grace	grade	grand	gradually
grain	grasp	gracious	gravely
grant	greet	gray	greatly
grape	grew	great	
grass	grieve	grateful	
grief	grip	green	
grin	groan	grim	
ground	grow		
group	growl		
grove	grown		
growth			
grandfather			
grandmother			
graduate			
gratitude			

Second Syllable Release

Nouns	Verbs	Adjectives
congress	agree	angry
degree		hungry
disgrace		Negro
program		
photograph		
telegram		
telegraph		

/kr/, Release

First Syllable Release

Nouns		Verbs	Adjectives
crew	crust	cry	crazy
cream	cradle	crack	cruel
creek	creature	crash	
crime	credit	crawl	
crop	critic	creep	
crow	crystal	crept	
crowd	creation	cross	
crown	criminal	crush	
crept		create	

Second and Third Syllable Release

Nouns	Verbs	Adjectives	Other
decrease	decrease	sacred	across
sacrifice		democratic	
secretary			
democrat			

/pr/, Release

First Syllable Release

Nouns	Verbs	Adjectives	Other
proof	pray	proud	presently
price	prove	pretty	probably
priest	preach	precious	practically
prize	press	practical	
praise	practice	previous	
present	pretend		
prison	prevent		
profit	promise		
problem	propose		
program	protect		
prophet	provide		
president			
protection			

Second Syllable Release

Nouns	Verbs	Adjectives
apron	approach	supreme
depression	approve	
impression	improve	
	appreciate	
	represent	

/tr/, Release

First Syllable Release

Nouns	Verbs
tree	try
trail	trace
train	track
tramp	trade
trap	treat
trial	travel
tribe	transfer
trick	tremble
truth	
traffic	
traitor	
treasure	
tribute	
trouble	
tragedy	
transportation	

Second and Third Syllable Release

Nouns	Verbs	Adjectives
contrast	attract	extra
country	betray	central
contract	control	electric
control	retreat	
distress	distribute	
entrance	introduce	
industry	illustrate	

/ər/, Release

First Syllable Release

Nouns	Verbs	Adjectives	Other
thrill	threw	three	through
throat	throw		
throne	thrust		
	threaten		

/s/ Blends

/sk/, Arrest

First Syllable Arrest

Nouns	Verbs
desk	ask
risk	risk
task	

/sk/, Release

First and Second Syllable Release

Nouns	Verbs	Adjectives
sky	scarce	scarce
scheme	score	
school	scorn	
score	skate	
scorn	sketch	
scout	escape	
sketch		
skill		
skin		
skirt		
basket		

/sm/, Release

First Syllable Release

Nouns	Verbs	Adjectives
smile	smile	small
smoke	smoke	smooth

/sn/, Release

First Syllable Release

Nouns	Verbs
snake	snap
snow	snatch

/sp/, Arrest

First Syllable Arrest

Nouns	Verbs
clasp	gasp
	grasp

/sp/, Release

First and Second Syllable Release

Nouns	Verbs	Adjectives
space	space	special
spark	spare	spoken
spear	spark	expensive
speech	speak	
speed	spill	
spoon	spend	
sport	spell	
spot	spin	
speaker	spare	
spider	spoil	
expert	spoke	
hospital	dispose	
	expect	

/st/, Arrest

First Syllable Arrest

Nouns		Verbs		Adjectives		Other
east	toast	boast	trust	east	vast	past
chest	vest	cost	twist	best	west	
host	west	lost		last	restless	
list	priest	must		next		
nest		rest				
post		taste				

Second Syllable Arrest

Nouns	Verbs		Adjectives	Other
forest	arrest	interest	earnest	against
breakfast	digest	invest	honest	almost
	distrust	protest	modest	utmost
	exhaust	suggest		
	insist			

/st/, Release

First Syllable Release

Nouns		Verbs		Adjectives
staff	stone	stage	store	steep
stage	stoop	stamp	startle	stern
stain	store	stand	stumble	stiff
stair	storm	stare		still
star	stove	start		stout
state	stable	stay		stuck
steam	standard	steal		stupid
stem	station	stop		steady
step	statue	sting		
sting	stomach	stir		
stock	story	stole		
	student	stood		
	study	stoop		
		stop		

Second and Third Syllable Release

Nouns	Verbs	Adjectives	Other
instinct	restore	instant	instead
costume	understand		
monster			
youngster			
institution			

/sw/, Release

First Syllable Release

Nouns	Verbs	Adjectives	Other
swamp	swarm	sweet	swiftly
swarm	sway	swift	
swim	swear		
swing	sweep		
	swell		
	swept		
	swim		
	swing		
	swallow		

BLENDS II

THREE-ELEMENT BLENDS

/spl/, Release

First Syllable Release

Verbs	Adjectives
splash	splendid
split	

/spr/, Release

First Syllable Release

Nouns	Verbs	Adjectives
spring	sprang	spry
	spread	
	sprinkle	

/str/, Release

First and Second Syllable Release

Nouns	Verbs	Adjectives	Other
straw	stretch	straw	strongly
stream	strike	strong	
street	struck	extra	
strip	struggle		
stroke			
string			
strength			
distress			

/skr/, Release

First Syllable Release

Nouns	Verbs
scratch	scratch
scream	scream
screech	screech
screen	screen
screw	screw

/skw/, Release

First Syllable Release

Nouns	Adjectives
squirrel	square
square	

BLENDS III

/t/, /d/, AND /w/ BLENDS

Most other blends appear too infrequently for extensive drill materials. However, some few lesser blends do appear with sufficient frequency in the English language so that drill lists would appear necessary. These lesser blends involve /t/, /d/, and /w/. Two-element blends with these sounds follow.

/t/ Blends

/nt/, Arrest

First Syllable Arrest

Nouns	Verbs	
ant	bent	paint
aunt	count	rent
cent	faint	sent
hint	hint	want
saint	mount	went
scent	pant	grant
tent		spent

Second Syllable Arrest

Nouns	Verbs	Adjectives
account	acquaint	absent
agent	appoint	brilliant
amount	consent	content
complaint	invent	different
event	prevent	gallant
extent		patient
giant		recent
infant		
intent		
moment		
parent		
present		

Third and Fourth Syllable Arrest

Nouns	Verbs	Adjectives
accident	represent	ignorant
amendment		innocent
apartment		
government		
monument		
president		
inhabitant		

/lt/, Arrest

First Syllable Arrest

Nouns	Verbs
belt	halt
bolt	built
colt	melt
fault	
salt	

Second Syllable Arrest

Nouns	Verbs
result	assault
revolt	

/kt/, Arrest

First Syllable Arrest

Nouns	Verbs
act	act
fact	

Second Syllable Arrest

Nouns	Verbs	Adjectives
subject	collect	direct
	contact	perfect
	elect	distinct

/pt/, Arrest

First Syllable Arrest

Verbs	Other
kept	promptly
wept	

Second and Third Syllable Arrest

Verbs
accept
adopt
interrupt

/ft/, Arrest

First Syllable Arrest

Nouns	Verbs	Adjectives
gift	left	left
	lift	soft

/d/ Blends

/nd/, Arrest

First Syllable Arrest

Nouns	Verbs	Adjectives	Other
end	bend	kind	and
band	find	round	kindly
bond	mend		
hound	mind		
land	send		
mind	tend		
pound	spend		
	stand		

Second Syllable Arrest

Nouns	Verbs	Adjectives	Other
diamond	attend	second	behind
errand	defend		
second	demand		
	intend		
	offend		
	remind		

/ld/, Arrest

First and Second Syllable Arrest

Nouns	Verbs	Adjectives	Other
child	build	old	behold
field	fold	bold	
gold	hold	cold	
mold	sold	gold	
world	told	mild	

/w/ Blends

/kw/, Release

First Syllable Release

Nouns	Verbs	Adjectives	Other
queen	quit	queer	quite
quarrel	quarrel	quick	quickly
quarter	quiver	quiet	
question			

/tw/, Release

First Syllable Release

Nouns	Verbs	Adjectives	Other
twig	twist	twelve	twice
twin		twenty	
twilight			
twinkle			

CONSONANTS AND BLENDS

MULTIPLE-FUNCTION CONSONANTS

Word lists follow in which consonants function in a multifaceted manner either to arrest and release the breath stream simultaneously or to arrest the breath stream in a word more than once or release the breath stream in a word more than once. A drill list involving words which contain more than one consonant blend appears after the consonant list.

/m/, Multiple Function

Nouns	Verbs	Adjectives	Other
meantime	murmur	medium	sometime
moment	memorize		
mushroom	remember		
museum			
amusement			
amendment			
management			
memory			
monument			

/n/, Multiple Function

Nouns	Verbs	Adjectives	Other
content	announce	nine	none
engine	concern	content	concerning
fountain	condemn	linen	
incline	confine	uncertain	
infant	consent	convenient	
linen	contain	innocent	
nation	convince	independent	
notion	intend	intelligent	
sunshine	invent	unfortunate	
attention	maintain		
conclusion	mention		
condition	continue		
connection	entertain		
convention	understand		
opinion			
ornament			
conversation			
information			
introduction			

/p/, Multiple Function

Nouns	Verbs	Adjectives	Other
pop	prepare	proper	properly
paper	propose	purple	
people			
pupil			
newspaper			
principal			
principle			
proportion			
proposal			
purpose			
population			
preparation			

/b/, Multiple Function

Nouns	Verbs
baby	absorb

/d/, Multiple Function

Nouns	Verbs	Adjectives	Other
dad	did	dead	indeed
deed	decide	dried	undoubtedly
candidate	divide	independent	
independence			

/k/, Multiple Function

Nouns	Verbs	Adjectives	Other
cake	cook	quick	quickly
clerk	kick	correct	
clock	conclude	chocolate	
cook	conduct	electric	
crack	connect		
critic	conquer		
conclusion			
consequence			

/t/, Multiple Function

Nouns	Verbs	Adjectives	Other
state	treat	stout	promptly
taste	trust	tight	instantly
tent	attract	straight	
test	construct	constant	
toast	protest	content	
treat	cultivate	important	
trust	disappoint	satisfactory	
contest	distribute		
contract	entertain		
contrast	hesitate		
ticket	interrupt		
title			
district			
intent			
patent			
retreat			
appetite			
apartment			
excitement			
gratitude			
investment			
multitude			
restaurant			
potato			
disappointment			
entertainment			
inhabitant			

/f/, Multiple Function

Nouns	Adjectives
photograph	fifth
philosophy	faithful
	fearful
	fifteen
	fifty

/v/, Multiple Function

Verbs	Adjectives
involve	velvet
survive	

/s/, Multiple Function

Nouns	Verbs	Adjectives	Other
sauce	assist	scarce	since
sense	consist	restless	seriously
absence	discuss	useless	
disgrace	dismiss	excellent	
disgust	exceed	expensive	
exhaust	insist	sensible	
exist	possess	serious	
expense	suggest	mysterious	
science	suspect	necessary	
sentence	suspend		
service	exercise		
silence			
success			
sunset			
surface			
assistance			
disaster			
exercise			
society			
experience			

/z/, Multiple Function

Nouns
disease
trousers

/tʃ/, Multiple Function

Nouns
church

/dʒ/, Multiple Function

Nouns
judge
judgment

/l/, Multiple Function

Nouns	*Adjectives*	*Other*
lily	level	largely
	helpless	lightly
	lively	absolutely
	little	silently
	lovely	slowly
	liberal	

/r/, Multiple Function

Nouns	*Verbs*	*Adjectives*	*Other*
roar	roar	rare	further
corner	murder	ordinary	rarely
order	order	primary	therefore
quarter	perform	regular	perfectly
record	prefer	particular	
reverse	prepare	extraordinary	
rider	record		
ruler	refer		
surprise	reform		
terror	restore		
treasure	retire		
emperor	return		
governor	reward		
grandfather	surprise		
grandmother	transfer		
property	transport		
treasury	recover		
restaurant			
corporation			
interior			
operator			

PHONEMIC CONTRASTS

Certain sounds are frequently confused with each other because auditory distinctions have not always been made between the sounds. It was mentioned earlier that distinctions may not be made between voiced and voiceless phonemes. The /w/ glide is substituted frequently for the consonant glide [r] and [l]. Phonemes produced by similar placement are frequently confused with each other. For example, /ə/ may be substituted for /s/, /ð/ for /z/, /s/ for /ʃ/, /p/ for [f]. Consonant types may be produced correctly as a group, but individual phonemes may be confused with each other. For example, plosives may be essentially mastered except for inconsistent substitution of /t/ for /k/ or vice versa. Front plosives /t/ and /d/ may be substituted for velar plosives. Even when one sound is not substituted for another and is produced correctly, error may occur with similar sounds made by similar placement. For example, some tongue tip consonants may be produced correctly while others may not be.

Word lists contrasting sounds frequently confused with each other may be very effective therapy because they stress auditory distinction between sounds which are confused with each other. Word lists contrasting sounds which are produced by similar placements can be effective when in the same list a sound produced correctly is contrasted with another sound which is produced incorrectly. For example, the child may elevate the tongue for /l/ but thrust it for /t/, and yet tongue elevation is necessary for both sounds. /s/ may be distorted while /ʃ/ is produced correctly, and yet the air stream passing over the tongue and cutting edge is necessary for both sounds. Word lists contrasting blends with consonants as singles may be very effective, because children may produce the sound correctly as a single but incorrectly as a blend, or correctly in a blend but incorrectly as a single.

Contrasting word lists differing only in the voicing dimension have already been presented, following word lists of individual phonemes. It will be apparent that many words in these lists are not from the fourth-grade reading level in Thorndike and Lorge. These additional words were added because relatively few words are available for the contrast lists in this source at this grade level. Other contrasts to be presented in the following pages are:

1. Plosive contrasts.

2. Placement contrasts, with word lists involving different phonemes produced by similar placements.

3. Auditory confusion contrasts, with word lists involving sounds which are frequently confused with each other.

4. Blend contrasts, with word lists involving consonants as single sounds and in blends.

PLOSIVE CONTRASTS

Contrasting Word Pairs Differing Only
with /t/ and /k/ Phonemes

/t/	/k/
tone	cone
top	cop
table	cable
take	cake
tap	cap
took	cook
told	cold
tall	call
tame	came
tan	can
too	coo
debt	deck
dot	dock
hat	hack
knot	knock
light	like
lot	lock
net	neck
oat	oak
pet	peck
pit	pick
rat	rack
rot	rock
rate	rake
ate	ache
bite	bike
lit	lick
might	mike
pat	pack
pet	peck
pit	pick
sit	sick
shot	shock
wait	wake
greet	Greek
hot	hock
but	buck
not	knock

Contrasting Word Pairs Differing Only
with /p/ and /t/ Phonemes

/p/	/t/
pea	tea
pie	tie
pack	tack
peach	teach
pear	tear
pen	ten
pile	tile
pin	tin
pop	top
paste	taste
porch	torch
pick	tick
ape	ate
cap	cat
cape	Kate
cup	cut
heap	heat
lip	lit
map	mat
nap	gnat
rope	wrote
sheep	sheet
soup	suit
top	tot
grip	grit
cheap	cheat
ripe	write

Contrasting Word Pairs Differing Only
with /p/ and /k/ Phonemes

/p/	/k/
ape	ache
cape	cake
lap	lack
lip	lick
nap	knack
shape	shake
sheep	sheik
sip	sick
tape	take
crop	crock
cheap	cheek
pea	key
page	cage
pain	cane
pear	care
pen	can
pin	kin
pit	kit
pole	coal
pot	cot
pat	cat

Contrasting Word Pairs Differing Only with /d/ and /g/ Phonemes

/d/	/g/
die	guy
dough	go
do	goo
dear	gear
down	gown
bed	beg
road	rogue
had	hag
lead	league
bad	bag
sad	sag

Contrasting Word Pairs Differing Only with /b/ and /g/ Phonemes

/b/	/g/
bag	gag
boat	goat
bold	gold
bun	gun
bus	Gus
bum	gum
by	guy
but	gut
robe	rogue
rub	rug

PLACEMENT CONTRASTS

Contrasting Word Pairs Differing Only
with /t/ and /l/ Phonemes

/t/	/l/
take	lake
tame	lame
tap	lap
tight	light
tip	lip
tuck	luck
tie	lie
tack	lack
Ted	led
tick	lick
took	look
toe	low
time	lime
tire	liar
toad	load
table	label
bought	ball
caught	call
fought	fall
ate	ale
eat	eel
boat	bowl
coat	coal
feet	feel
foot	full
gate	gale
goat	goal
hate	hail
heat	heel
meat	meal
rate	rail
fight	file
fit	fill
hit	hill
meat	meal

/t/ (cont.)	/l/ (cont.)
pat	pal
put	pull
sit	sill
fate	fail
neat	kneel
wet	well
it	ill

Contrasting Words Differing Only with /p/, /b/, and /m/ Phonemes

/p/	/b/	/m/
pea	be	me
pie	buy	my
pat	bat	mat
path	bath	math
pass	bass	mass
pan	ban	man
pen	Ben	men
pit	bit	mitt
pail	bail	mail
park	bark	mark
puff	buff	muff
cup	cub	come
rip	rib	rim
rope	robe	roam

Contrasting Words Differing Only with /t/, /d/, /l/, and /n/ Phonemes

/t/	/d/	/l/	/n/
toe	dough	low	no
tie	die	lie	nigh
at	add	Al	an
cat	cad	Cal	can
coat	code	coal	cone
bet	bed	bell	Ben
mate	made	mail	main

AUDITORY CONFUSION CONTRASTS

Contrasting Words Differing Only with /w/, Consonant
Glide [r], and Semivowel [l] Phonemes

/w/	[r]	[l]
way	ray	lay
wake	rake	lake
weed	read	lead
week	reek	leak
weight	rate	late
weep	reap	leap
went	rent	lent
wink	rink	link
wise	rise	lies
why	rye	lie
white	right	light
where	rare	lair

Contrasting Word Pairs Differing Only
with the /p/ and /f/ Phonemes

/p/	/f/
plea	flea
pig	fig
pile	file
pin	fin
pit	fit
paint	faint
pat	fat
pour	four
pull	full
put	foot
pale	fail
cap	calf
whip	whiff
wipe	wife
cheap	chief
picks	fix
picked	fixed

Contrasting Word Pairs Differing Only with /s/ and /θ/ or /ð/ Phonemes

/s/	/θ/, /ð/
sank	thank
see	thee
sing	thing
sat	that
sick	thick
seem	theme
sin	thin
sew	though
some	thumb
sis	this
face	faith
saw	thaw
sum	thumb
sat	that
sis	this
sail	they'll

Contrasting Word Pairs Differing Only with /ʃ/ and /tʃ/ Phonemes

/ʃ/	/tʃ/
shoe	chew
sheep	cheap
sheet	cheat
ship	chip
shop	chop
share	chair
she's	cheese
sheik	cheek
shin	chin
sheer	cheer
shoes	choose
sherry	cherry
dish	ditch
crush	crutch
wash	watch
wish	witch
mash	match
cash	catch
mush	much

Contrasting Word Pairs Differing Only with /s/ and /tʃ/ Phonemes

/s/	/tʃ/
seat	cheat
sat	chat
seek	cheek
seize	cheese
sink	chink
soak	choke
sick	chick
sicken	chicken
sore	chore
shoes	choose
shows	chose

Contrasting Word Pairs Differing Only with /s/ and /ʃ/ Phonemes

/s/	/ʃ/
see	she
sea	she
sack	shack
seat	sheet
seed	she'd
sign	shine
son	shun
suit	shoot
said	shed
save	shave
seek	sheik
seize	she's
sell	shell
sew	show
same	shame
sore	shore
so	show
gas	gash
class	clash
brass	brash

Two-Element Blends and Single-Sound Contrasts

/sk/ Blend Words Divided into Words Containing /k/ and /s/ Phonemes

/sk/	/k/	/s/
scale		sale
scheme		seem
school	cool	
score	core	sore
scorn	corn	
skate	Kate	
skill	kill	sill
skin	kin	sin
sky		sigh
scare	care	

/st/ Blend Words Divided into Words Containing /s/ and /t/ Phonemes

/st/	/t/	/s/
stair	tear	
stake	take	sake
star	tar	
stalk	talk	
steam	team	seem
steel		seal
stick	tick	sick
stock	tock	sock
stoop		soup
stone	tone	
stun	ton	sun
stop	top	
store	tore	sore

/sl/ Blend Words Divided into Words
Containing /s/ and /l/ Phonemes

/sl/	/s/	/l/
sleep		leap
sleeve		leave
slice		lice
slide	side	lied
slip	sip	lip
slain		lain
slay	say	lay
slight	sight	light
slender	sender	lender

/cl/ Blend Words Divided into Words
Containing /k/ and /l/ Phonemes

/cl/	/k/	/l/
clean		lean
clock	cock	lock
clay		lay
clues		lose
clamp	camp	lamp
claim	came	lame
clam		lamb
clap	cap	lap
class		lass
claw		law
click	kick	lick
clip		lip
clot	cot	lot
cloud		loud
cluck		luck

3. Treatment for Articulation Disorder

The sections which follow will deal with treatment for the child with an articulation disorder. Two differing methods of evaluation and treatment which are used widely will be considered. Finally, the author will suggest a third method which borrows some principles from these two methods. The author believes that his method will result in improvement of articulation over relatively short periods of time, and has found, at least in his own experience, that it reduces the percentage of time spent in repetitive drill. The speech materials found in the previous section will form the basis for the speech therapy techniques to be proposed. A rationale will be described which is based on normative data concerning the patterning children apparently follow in mastering the phonological dimension of speech.

ASSESSMENT OF ARTICULATION

Adequate assessment of consonant articulation as single phonemes and blends needs to precede any recommendations for speech training of a child with an articulation disorder. Phonemic errors can be classified according to three main types: (1) omissions, referring to leaving off of sounds in words; (2) distortions, referring to substandard or unclear production of sounds; and (3) substitutions, referring to productions of phonemes which are different from the intended phonemes. Articulation errors are classified further according to their position or location within the test words (Van Riper, 1965).

Tests

Two picture articulation tests widely used for the nonreader are the Developmental Articulation Test (1959) and the Templin-Darley Tests of Articulation (1960). Both tests assess production of individual consonants and blends as the child names specific pictures. The first test involves 78 consonant phonemes, 64 as singles and 14 in double blends. The test has a severe limitation: there are few blend items. When a child has articulation difficulty, blends will usually be involved, and can be an excellent starting point for speech therapy, as a later section will indicate. The test does not consider the degree of consistency of the error, another major weakness.

The Templin-Darley Tests are more comprehensive. The tests consist of 176 items: 12 vowels, 6 diphthongs, 68 consonants as singles, 37 consonants in double blends, 16 consonants in triple blends, 23 [r] vowel items, and 14 [l] vowel items.

The Templin-Darley Tests seek to measure the degree of consistency by including items in which sounds may be listed which are produced correctly as blends but incorrectly as singles, or, vice versa, sounds which are produced incorrectly as blends but correctly as singles. An item is included also for listing sounds often produced incorrectly as singles but produced correctly as singles in at least one position in some test words. For sounds which are consistently produced incorrectly, there is an item to denote those sounds which were produced correctly following strong auditory stimulation. The placement of the blends and the arrangement of the test form make completion difficult, and interpretation of the data is very time consuming.

Templin and Darley suggest in these tests the use of questions and statements printed on the backs of the picture cards in order to avoid monotonous repetition of the question "What is this?" Spoken questions can indeed unduly delay administration of the test and negatively affect the motivation of the child. However, children will usually name the stimulus picture without the use of questions or remarks. Furthermore, articulation results can be invalidated if the child does not have the experiential background to understand the stimulus remark. For example: (1) The test word for initial /b/ is *bear*, and the stimulus remark is "This is Smoky the _____." (2) The test word for medial /d/ is *wading*, and the stimulus remark is "The boys aren't swimming. They're _____." (3) The test word for final /s/ is *mouse*, and the stimulus remark is "Hickory-dickory-dock. The _____ ran up the clock."

Both tests classify errors according to the three types previously noted: omissions, distortions, and substitutions. Both tests use a positional classification to specify the place of the error in the test word. The error is either in the initial position of the test word, the first sound in the word, the medial position in the test word, occurring within the word, or the final position, the last sound of the test word. The majority of sounds can occur in all three positions, but a few consonants can occur in only two positions. Only three blends, /sp/, /st/, and /sk/, out of more than 150 occur in all three positions, while other blends occur in only one or two positions (Fries, 1963). The positional classification of consonant errors has previously been described as artificial. Therapy based on the positional scheme tends to prolong training time unduly, as will be discussed in the articulation treatment later.

A recently developed articulation test, "A Deep Test of Articulation," strongly condemns positional classification, and identifies phonemes as functioning elements in a syllable to either release, shape, or arrest the syllable (McDonald, 1964A, 1964B, 1964C). Words are made up of one or more syllables with individual sounds "appearing as overlapping movements superimposed on the syllable." Sounds are "studied as parts of movement sequences rather than as positions in words." In the picture form of this test, when an articulation error is found, two different sets of picture cards are used simultaneously to "deep" test the sound in a variety of phonetic contexts, as the sound is preceded and followed by vowels, and as the sound is followed and preceded by each of the other consonants. The dimension of consonant error inconsistency is thus probed very thoroughly in the test. By sampling consonant production in many phonetic contexts, one will generally find a phonetic context in which the error sound is produced correctly.

In the "deep" testing of the consonant /s/, for example, as it is preceded by other consonants, the child names the individual pictures in one set, combining each name with the word *sun* pictured in the second set. Care is taken to prevent the child from pausing between naming of the pictures so that the articulators do not return to a "physiologic rest position." The child constructs the following "funny words" *cupsun, tubsun, kitesun,* etc. Notation is made on an individual test blank of the kind of consonant production in each phonetic context: correct, omission error, distortion error, or substitution error.

The test makes a significant contribution in the field of articulation testing and therapy because of the emphasis on inconsistency of phoneme production, and because this is used as a basis for subsequent therapy. Emphasis is placed on the function of the consonant and the consistency of the consonant error in extended speech utterances of the child in many different phonetic contexts, thereby providing information which may not be secured from more conventional tests which base their results on phonemic production in isolated words.

However, the test has some severe limitations. It can be extremely long and laborious. This author cannot "deep test" more than two sounds at one meeting if they are evaluated in all phonetic contexts. The results are not valid for children with certain types of speech problems. The author has found, for example, that children who speak slowly and children with multiple articulation errors have difficulty blending the two separate words into one single word without pausing. Yet these children do not have these difficulties in speaking when pauses are part of natural speaking situations. Children with neuromuscular disorders involving the articulators have trouble also in joining words without a pause, particularly when fricatives are blended together. They are not able to make the articulatory adjustments necessary to produce all the "funny words" in the test. The construction of "funny words" can provoke too much laughter and thus reduce motivation. Some children may even resist saying the words because of these reactions and thus negate validity of any test results. When the author assigned the test for use by experienced therapists pursuing graduate work in speech pathology, the therapists were very critical of their findings. They felt that many hours of listening to the responses of children to the test items would be necessary before they could consider their findings to be valid.

The Fairbanks tests (Fairbanks, 1960) are used widely, one test for the primary reader and another test for the child who is a better reader. The Deep Test of Articulation (McDonald, 1964B, 1964C) has two forms, the picture form and written sentence form. As with the picture test, with the sentence test two different sets of sentences are used, one set for the consonant preceded by a vowel and other consonants immediately following, and the second set for the consonant followed by the vowel and other consonants immediately preceding, the consonant being "deep tested." The Templin-Darley Tests (1960) also have two forms, with the written sentence form testing the same sounds as the picture form.

ARTICULATION TREATMENT

The particular method used for treating children with articulation errors follows from the rationale and findings of the articulation assessment. Those who evaluate articulation errors in terms of position use an approach which is different from those who evaluate the error in terms of movement sequences. This section will describe both approaches. Finally, a third approach used with success by the author will be suggested, based in part on certain aspects of both approaches. This third approach bases its rationale on findings which deal with the way normal-speaking children develop in their acquisition of articulation skills.

STIMULATION METHOD

Clinicians who assess articulation according to a three-positional system use the so-called stimulation method to teach correct production of the error sound in all three positions in words. The child producing the sound incorrectly is believed not to hear the differences between the correct production of the phoneme and his incorrect production. Therefore the child needs first to recognize through hearing alone the differences between error and correct production of the phoneme before any attempts are made to correct the production. Van Riper and Irwin (1958) believe the tactual and kinesthetic feedback systems are in control with the child having articulation errors. The auditory modality needs to regain the dominance which it had when the child was first learning to speak. The child needs to be able to identify incorrect phonemic production and correct phonemic production in the speech of others ("interpersonal auditory circuit"). He needs to recognize the error in his own speech ("intrapersonal auditory circuit"). "The intrapersonal (self-hearing) and interpersonal (hearing the therapist) circuits must be brought into resonance. They must harmonize" (Van Riper, and Irwin, 1958, page 139). Correct production of the sound cannot be taught until the child is able first to identify and contrast incorrect and correct productions of the sound or sounds which he produces incorrectly. Teaching of correct production begins after the person can discriminate between error and nonerror. Correct sound production involves a blended feedback from three sensory circuits, tactual, kinesthetic, and auditory.

The so-called stimulation or stimulus method is the training procedure used with the positional system for analysis of the articulation error. The system is logical and reasonable, starting at the earliest level of speech and teaching with total emphasis on the auditory modality for the initial step. Sound production is introduced in the simplest phonetic context. Drill materials involving more complicated phonetic contexts are introduced before mastery of correct production is sought in habitual speech. The stimulation method employs the following six discrete steps in the therapeutic process:

1. Auditory identification of the correct and incorrect production of the sound in the speech of others and in the speech of the person receiving speech training.

2. Production of the sound in isolation.

3. Production of the sound in nonsense syllables in terms of the three positions, initial, medial, and final.

4. Production of the sound in drill words in terms of the three positions.

5. Production of drill words in sentences and paragraphs.

6. Carry-over of correct production of sound into nucleus social situations and finally into habitual speech (Johnson et al., 1967; Van Riper, 1965).

Numerous games are employed in each of the six steps to make the tasks pleasing to the child. For example, games for auditory discrimination, the first step, include hiding games, with the clinician producing the sound correctly when the child is near the hidden object and producing the sound incorrectly when the child is far from the hidden object. Or material is read aloud to the child, with the drill sound spoken either correctly or incorrectly. When the clinician produces the sound correctly, the child responds with one signal, such as raising the right hand or touching the right ear. When the clinician produces the sound incorrectly, the child responds with another signal, such as raising the left hand or touching the left ear.

When the child begins work on production of the sound, a multitude of games are available commercially involving ladders to ascend with correct production and descend with incorrect production; spinners and boards with stops on the spinners being the drill sound and movement on the board being allowed only with correct production; lotto games with pictures of objects containing the drill sound which the child may place on the master card when production is correct but not when production is incorrect. Games of concentration, similar to the television program, use paired pictures containing the drill sound; if the child remembers the positional location of the sound and produces correctly he is able to keep the picture, but if he produces incorrectly he is not allowed to keep the picture even if he remembers the location.

A month does not pass without mail coming at least twice to the speech clinician advertising games for various sounds either as singles or blends. There is the racing game for the /r/, the baseball game for the /s/, the fishing game for the /f/, and the shooting game for /ʃ/, etc. Correction of a particular sound suggests a particular game. The rules of the game are usually very simple, but all are designed to make speech "fun." While the games are supposedly secondary to speech and utilized only to make speech training a pleasant learning experience, experience suggests that the games become of more importance to the child than the speech. The games and desire to win become so important that the child forgets the reason for his attending speech classes. When speech is used during the games, the amount and kind of speech become secondary to the importance of the game. Speech therapy is conceived of as the speech involved in playing games and not as a means of social exchange and communication of ideas and feelings. When asked the purpose and activities of going to "speech class," children will frequently state they "play games." If pressed, they may conceivably remember that particular sounds are involved in the game activities.

The clinician may well have told the children that the purposes of their meetings are for improved speech, but for the child the game activities are the purposes. Those children who like games and conceive of them as a means of being excused from academic classes will look forward to speech therapy. Those children who do not like games and enjoy academic classes will not like speech therapy because they may believe they are not working on correcting speech.

In such circumstances, results from speech therapy can well be reduced and protracted, leading to increased numbers of children on waiting lists. If speech therapy involves speech which is required and necessary for learning and social activities, results will be faster and quicker. There is no apparent reason for disguising the purposes of and need for improved speech. Children usually know well enough the shame, embarrassment, and social discomfort which result from poor speech. In his fantasy world many a child with defective speech pictures himself as a great orator, lawyer, statesman, or politician delivering momentous speeches to large crowds who are eager to hear every spoken word.

Children learn mathematics by doing math, they learn to read by reading, and they should learn to speak by speaking. The aim of this book is to present carefully selected and organized speech materials which are designed for speech activities. Games are not viewed as undesirable per se, but rather are viewed as pleasant activities which can involve speech if the game can be truly relegated to a position of secondary importance. They should be regarded as one activity among many for speech involvement, or they may be viewed as a reward after intensive drill work on speech. If this second way of using games is followed, then sounds are not drilled on, phoneme production is not evaluated, and the game is played for fun only.

In the same way, literature should be viewed as something to be enjoyed for its own sake. How many stories and poems are read aloud with the child attending to production of specific phonemes, the "how" of speaking, and not the content, the beauty of language, the "what" of speaking? Literature should, of course, be used during speech therapy to illustrate the beauty of language. Speech activity involved in oral reading is intended for appreciation of the quality of the writing; it should not superficially relegate literature to a position of less importance than the number of /s/ phonemes spoken correctly by the child or teacher. A later section will detail the kinds of speech activities which can be used with success during speech therapy.

Numerous times previously it has been mentioned that articulation errors are generally inconsistent and that detailed testing of error sounds will usually reveal instances in which the sound is produced correctly. Three of the six steps listed under "Stimulation Method" appear unnecessary in the light of this evidence. The "intrapersonal auditory circuit" and the "interpersonal auditory circuit" would appear to be in "resonance" during the instances of correct production. The auditory feedback system of the child with an articulation disorder is apparently no different from that of other speakers, at least during the times of correct production.

Thus the isolation of the sound with excessive ear training before the child is allowed to produce the sound in any phonetic context involves an excessive amount of unnecessary time. Further, a consonant can never be produced in isolation. As soon as a consonant releases the breath stream a vowel is released also. Stetson (1951) concludes, therefore, that the syllable is the smallest unit into which a consonant can be divided for speech purposes. If the child is already able to produce the sound correctly in some words, he can begin immediately with whole words in articulation training, step 4 as previously outlined, and proceed to complete mastery of the sound through the steps following. Spriestersbach and Curtis (1951) discuss the inconsistency of articulation errors in the speech of children in the early elementary grades as reported in numerous studies. However, they conclude from these findings that all the steps in the stimulation method are necessary but that ear training, step 1, should begin with those phonetic environments in which production is correct. They write that ear training "adapted to the particular phonetic context in which the individual's misarticulations occur is probably more effective than the gross type now commonly employed" (page 49).

Powers (1957) talks also of the consistency of articulation errors and states that "some individuals make the acoustic errors consistently. . . . Others vary greatly, using the sound correctly in some words, omitting it in others and using substitutions for it in others. It is not uncommon for a sound which occurs twice within one word to be given differently in the two positions" (page 712). She stresses the need for a thorough evaluation of the specific sounds and the phonetic contexts in which errors on the sounds occur. However, Powers also begins training with auditory discrimination without starting at the articulation level of the child.

Holland (1967) talks of "progressive approximation and shaping" in programming for children with articulation errors. Considerable interest exists in developing automated programs, with the idea that correction of errors may be achieved over a shorter period of time, and that fewer clinicians will be needed since the machine alone can regulate the development and sequencing of material. Programming might be of value for the child with consistent articulation errors whose auditory system is so deficient that he is unable to identify his error via the auditory channel. It has been pointed out that the majority of children with articulation errors produce the sounds correctly in some phonetic context. If, then, responses are already correct in some contexts, there would appear to be no need for "approximations." Where programming is developed, one needs to be very careful to build a program around the individual needs of a particular child. Observations suggest that frequently a child is made to fit into an existing program without the careful regard for his articulation needs and strengths.

Further, children with articulation difficulty may experience considerable pain and discomfort in speaking to people and may seek to avoid speaking situations whenever possible. When these children realize that they can speak to the clinician, however, without emotional anguish, and that the clinician is able to understand them without severe effort, they may well be rewarded sufficiently to try speech with others.

In a manner of speaking, this is analogous to a child with a severe behavioral disorder who has considerable difficulties in relating to his peers and adults. As, however, he finds comfort and security in relating to one other person, he then becomes daring and seeks to relate to other persons. Similarly, as children with articulation difficulties experience continued success in their daily speaking, they may well be motivated to excellent accomplishments. The machine hardly affords the humanness and warmth of approach which persons with speaking difficulties may need.

ARTICULATION MOVEMENT SEQUENCES

This method uses the context in which the sound is produced correctly, as discovered by the "deep test," as the starting point for articulation therapy. Therapy begins first with those sequences in which the sound is produced correctly and extends to other phonetic contexts in which the sound is produced incorrectly. Unlike the stimulation method, which uses only the auditory modality, particularly during beginning therapy, the articulation movement sequence method uses all learning modalities—proprioceptive, tactile, and auditory—from the beginning. All sensory input systems are immediately integrated in the learning of correct articulation.

The actual procedure, however, appears to obscure the consistency-inconsistency phenomenon so that the child lacks awareness of the factors accounting for the sometimes correct, sometimes incorrect production. When a "movement sequence" results in correct production, the child cannot know the reason for variable articulation, one instance correct and another instance incorrect, because he needs to continue speaking, not being given pause time to reflect on the differences in production. The "movement sequences" per se during speech are too many, too different, and too complex to understand. Different articulators moving in different ways account for the different productions, but the movements are far too numerous to analyze during speaking, particularly if time is not allotted to analysis and discussions concerning speech and what we do when we are talking.

Overlapping speech sounds are used in testing and therapy rather than discrete sounds because speakers use overlapping movements in speech, with the result that sounds can influence other sounds dependent on the phonetic contexts in which they appear. Further, no English phoneme is the same in all phonetic environments "though in many phonemes the variations can easily be overlooked" (Gleason, 1961, page 258). McDonald (1964A, page 85) therefore states: "There obviously cannot be an individual speech sound which is always the same. We don't have a [k] sound but rather we have [k] sounds. There are as many [k] sounds as there are phonetic contexts because each phonetic context requires a different pattern of overlapping movements." McDonald recognizes that there are 1225 contexts in which /k/ might appear, but tests for only "approximately 50 phonetic contexts" in the "deep test." There are obviously many phonetic contexts still unsampled in the test. Speech movements, the basis of this approach, are highly variable for the productions of any single phoneme. The movements possible for any sound are too numerous to sample. "There is no such thing as a definite group of speech movements uniformly repeated or successive pronunciation of the 'same letter'" (Shohara, 1964, page 21). Since movement as such can never be repeated exactly, it becomes impossible to adapt this scheme for clinical speech training. Stetson comments, however, that "movement of sounds often overlap and often fuse; they are not always separate. The syllable is always a separate event in the speech series and while investigators may not find it easy to determine the principle of syllable division, no one has assumed that two syllables could in any sense overlap or coincide" (page 27). Articulation training, then, could well start with the syllable before involving it in phonetic contexts in which there is overlapping speech.

The use of "overlapping movements" in syllable drill appears to offer no significant advantage, clinically, over handling the phonemic error in terms of the location of the error in words as is practiced by the stimulation method. The Pennsylvania rationale (McDonald, 1964B, 1964C) while abandoning the tedious process of drilling on consonants in terms of a three-positional orientation, has substituted a procedure involving "movement sequences" which are equally, if not more, tedious and time consuming. Speech materials involved in training are artificial, as a later example will illustrate. In addition, the choice of representative movements for training is difficult, as is the decision concerning the number and kinds of movements. A single movement is never repeated, as has been discussed, and thus the universe of possible movements is apparently infinite. Both clinician and patient are certain to be frustrated by the inability to find starting or ending points.

To illustrate the application of this method, McDonald (1964A) cites a young child who misarticulates the /s/ in many phonetic contexts but who produces the /s/ correctly on the picture Deep Test when it was preceded by /tʃ/ and followed by /ʌ/ in the movement sequence for the "funny word" *watchsun*. Sentence dialogue is "introduced" (page 145):

CLINICIAN: Did you say, "Look, sun will burn you"?
CHILD: No, I said, "Watch, sun will burn you."
CLINICIAN: Did you say, "Watch, fire will burn you"?
CHILD: No, I said, "Watch, sun will burn you."
CLINICIAN: Did you say, "Watch, sun might burn you"?
CHILD: No, I said, "Watch, sun will burn you."
CLINICIAN: Did you say, "Watch, sun will tan you"?
CHILD: No, I said, "Watch, sun will burn you."

Although the "funny word" used in extended speech supposedly represents a specific movement involving /s/, each production of the word will involve a different movement for the sound (Shohara, 1964). The dialogue and vocabulary are very contrived despite attempts to simulate actual speech. How many children will be successful in using this kind of dialogue? Children of early elementary school age would lack the linguistic facility for such a verbal exchange. The older child is interested in using speech as a tool for expressing ideas and feelings. It seems doubtful that this dialogue fulfills the need of using speech for communication. Such an approach and vocabulary will not be acceptable for the majority of adults.

The writer wonders how comfortable clinicians are with this kind of dialogue. The clinician who feels uncomfortable cannot be natural and warm with children. When the relationship is not warm, results emerging from the relationship will no doubt suffer.

If a child or adult can produce the /s/ correctly in the fabricated word *watchsun*, he is probably able to produce the sound correctly in the word *sun*. By attending to tongue placement and occlusal relationships for correct production, he will probably be able to produce the sound correctly in other words of one syllable in which /s/ releases the syllable and is followed by the neutral vowel /ʌ/. Such words as *sun, such, suck, sup* could be tried. If the /s/ is distorted in either of the words, the probable reason is that the sound arresting the syllable has an effect on the sound which releases the syllable. Drill can immediately involve actual words, with discussion centering on speech which is involved in production of actual words.

For a child receiving speech therapy, the strongest motivating device is improvement in saying words which the adults in his environment have tried to help him say. By isolating words in which production of a sound is already correct, the child is motivated to try other words in which production of the sound is incorrect. Production of sounds in a multitude of nonsense syllables will have little or no meaning to a child. Continuous repetition of the meaningless syllables in contrived dialogue can prove monotonous and unmotivating to many children. They do not understand the purpose of the drills, and the words are not the language they use or which they hear others use. However, if the child can produce the sound correctly in actual words, the learning becomes meaningful. As he finds himself able to produce the sound correctly in more words, he derives early benefits from speech therapy and he consequently becomes highly motivated and involved in the learning process. While the phenomenon of inconsistency of phonemic production serves as a basis for articulation therapy with the movement sequence method, the actual procedure and materials do not begin at the word level; in the forced concern for overlapping movements, therapy materials are actually disguised nonsense syllables, conceivably step 3 in the stimulation method. Many children may find the procedures and materials unmotivating. Clinicians may be uncomfortable using the method and are likely to have a difficult time securing and utilizing materials.

WHOLE WORD METHOD OF ASSESSMENT AND TREATMENT

The author believes that articulation evaluation should explore the realm of inconsistency of phonemic production in actual words, units meaningful, understandable, and important to the speaker with poor articulation. Those words in which the phoneme is produced correctly are used immediately in the whole word method of articulation training. The words in which phonemic production is correct are compared with words in which phonemic production is incorrect.

For the child with an articulation disorder, the phoneme is the unit which needs to be mastered consistently in all words. It can be considered first, generally speaking, in one-syllable words in which there is no overlapping speech movement, and later in polysyllabic words and in multiple word contexts involving pauses, stresses, and varieties of overlapping movements. Naming or one-word answers to questions are among the kinds of materials which require one-word answers. Extended responses may then be developed from these one-word responses, with the clinician noting carefully those phonetic environments which are easiest. The words, whether in single units or in phrases of varying length, need to become part of a communicative situation which involves a speaker and listener. Speech materials need to fit naturally in a social situation involving speech. The ultimate aim of mastery of all phonemes in all words and in all types of speaking situations gradually becomes possible as mastery of more sounds is realized in more phonetic contexts involved in more speaking situations.

Level of phonemic mastery will need to be explored first in the single-word responses before phonemic production is explored in longer units which involve syntactical elements and overlapping movements, both of which influence phonemic production. There is abundant conclusive evidence to indicate that, while young children produce phonemes incorrectly in some words, they will produce the same phoneme correctly in other words. Irwin (1947A, 1947B) found that all consonant phonemes are acquired by 2½ years of age with the exception of the affricates /dʒ/ and /tʒ/. Lewis (1951) notes that 81 per cent of substitution errors involve sounds already produced by very young children.

As the child becomes older, the percentage of his incorrect production becomes less. For example, four sounds frequently mentioned as being incorrectly produced by young children are /s/, /ʃ/, /z/, and /tʃ/ (Fairbanks, 1960). The results of Templin's cross-sectional study (1957, pages 162–163), using a positional classification with children presumably without speech defects, are demonstrated in Table 1. In the process of acquiring complete mastery of the four sounds shown in Table 1, some children with normal speech produce these sounds correctly in some words when they are as young as three years old. While more children produce the sounds correctly at the terminal age of eight, some have not mastered production of these four phonemes in all words by the age of eight. While the speech of particular children is not described by the above table, it is

TABLE 1. Number of Subjects Out of Total of 60 at Each Age Level Who Correctly Articulate Sounds Shown*

Sound	3	3–5	4	4–5	5	6	7	8
s-	42	51	46	48	47	46	55	58
-s-	39	49	46	45	47	43	53	57
-s	35	41	44	46	46	47	53	56
sh-	32	43	45	53	52	52	57	59
-sh-	24	32	37	47	44	52	57	57
-sh	24	38	45	52	52	52	57	58
z-	18	33	37	43	39	40	54	57
-z-	28	45	43	45	45	47	54	57
-z	15	21	25	30	32	29	47	45
ch-	30	36	43	45	49	53	59	57
-ch-	28	38	44	52	51	53	57	58
-ch	26	35	42	53	52	50	56	58

* Reprinted by permission from Templin (1957).

highly probable that those children of seven and eight years producing one of these four sounds defectively in the initial position are different from those of like age producing the sound defectively in the other positions. The maturational process involving consonant mastery suggests that sounds are mastered gradually at different times in different phonetic contexts until the sound is mastered in all phonetic contexts. While the children are learning to master all consonant phonemes in the language, they are speaking words and, either alone or with the help of adults in the environment, learning to master all consonant phonemes.

If children with normal articulation growth undergo this patterning on their way to consonant mastery, children who are presumably slower in growth toward normal articulation can be helped toward consonant mastery by utilizing these same materials. Specialists in child development (Olson, 1959) point out that children go through the same patterning in their growth and maturational process, but that rates of growth differ. In sequential development leading to walking, for example, children generally first sit up, crawl, stand with assistance, stand without assistance, walk with assistance, and walk without assistance. Within this patterning, some children become earlier walkers than others and, conversely, some children become later walkers than others. In the area of speech development, articulation also shows differing rates of growth, just as does motor development. All children can be expected to follow the pattern of inconsistency of articulation production before consonant mastery, regardless of their rate of mastery.

Normal-speaking children may be expected to master articulation during the eighth year of life except for occasional incorrect production of fricatives, affricates, or blends. Children of kindergarten and first grade age can therefore be expected to produce some consonant sounds incorrectly. As a matter of fact, it would be the rule rather than the exception that the speech of the average child in these grades would contain consonant errors (Roe and Milisen, 1942). Even so, there will be other children who will achieve consonant mastery before they are eight years of age, and children with articulation difficulty who will have articulation errors when they are older than eight. Observations of the speech of intellectually normal children of early elementary school age will provide ample evidence of the individual differences in their speech behavior. Some children will achieve consonant mastery quicker than other children, and conversely some children will achieve consonant mastery later than other children.

When the articulation evaluation indicates that the child is retarded significantly in terms of age expectations, articulation therapy can be recommended. The child of kindergarten age may not be in need of therapy if one or several fricatives and blends are produced incorrectly. However, the child should be intelligible despite the presence of these errors. If the child is unintelligible or if great effort is required for understanding, speech therapy is recommended for the child of kindergarten age, particularly if he is developing fears and anxieties when called on to speak in the class-room. Speech therapy would not be indicated for the child in the first and second grades if the fricative errors are inconsistent, indicating the be-ginning of mastery, but an apparently consistent error involving a particu-lar fricative may indicate the need for therapy. If several consonant errors are involved in the speech of a child in the first or second grade, speech therapy may be indicated dependent on the intelligibility of the child, the consistency of the error, and the psychological effect of the errors on the social adjustment of the youngster. A child in the third grade who is advancing normally in all other motor skills and school subjects should be expected to master all phonemes and two-element blends except for a very occasional error by the time a child is in the third grade. If consonant errors are present in the speech of the child in the third grade, speech therapy should be recommended (Goda, 1970).

A distinction needs to be made between the speech problem of mis-pronunciation and that of an articulation disorder. If a certain sound is produced incorrectly in only one or a few specific words, but correctly in all other words, the speech problem is one of mispronunciation and not an articulation disorder. An articulation disorder by definition involves mis-production of a phoneme or phonemes in specific phonetic contexts.

The author has seen children who were receiving therapy for an articula-tion disorder but who proved to have errors only in the pronunciation of certain specific words. Speech therapy will be prolonged and relatively ineffective if training centers on phonemic mastery in phonetic contexts when the child's errors involve mispronunciation. As an example, a third grade child was brought by the mother to a hospital speech and hearing clinic because of omissions of the /t/ phoneme. Speech therapy was recommended by the school therapist, but her schedule was too full for new cases. Evaluation revealed that omissions occurred only with these specific frequently appearing words: *let, can't,* and *put.* The sound was produced in all other words. The omission errors were handled by considering the specific words only as discrete units and in extended utterances. Extended drills and mastery of the phoneme in different phonetic contexts was not indi-cated, as they would be with an articulation error. Young children of four, five, and even six years may omit entire syllables in polysyllabic words, yet their articulation is acceptable for their age. The children may lack practice in producing words which involve three or more syllables. There-fore they may omit the syllables, because the auditory feedback system has not as yet been developed to include many words of three or more syllables.

As examples, in the speech of such a child the words *superintendent* and *hippopotamus* may lack one or two syllables and articulation may involve faulty blending. Shorter words such as *hospital, principal,* and *gymnasium* may be spoken without all the syllables. Stress may be faulty in polysyllabic words because primary, secondary, and tertiary stress are necessary. Several syllables may receive the primary stress or equal secondary stress. Corrective work, if necessary, should stress polysyllabic words in therapy, with attention directed to developing auditory feedback to include all syllables in a word.

Children with linguistic deficiencies may omit specific phonemes, but this error results from inadequate knowledge of the morphemes in the English language. If the child does not know the rules for forming plurals, he will omit the plural morpheme and thus the three allomorphs /-s/, /-z/, /-ɪz/ (Baratz, 1969). Further listening to the speech of the child is necessary in order to determine if the error involves the phoneme /s/ or /z/ or whether it is specific with linguistic deficiency. If the latter is the cause, training needs to involve teaching of the rules for plurals without involvement of articulation.

ASSESSMENT OF ARTICULATION

When speech therapy is recommended, the therapy prescribed should have as a frame of reference the patterning of the child who is not retarded in consonant mastery. Therapy utilizing whole words and development of consistent mastery from inconsistent mastery should thus be the basis of materials selected for articulation teaching.

All children with articulation disorders have similarities in that each has phonemic errors during speaking. However, each child has his unique pattern of articulation development involving the consistency of his errors. While an occasional child will have articulation errors which are consistent, the average child has articulation errors which are inconsistent. Treatment for an articulation disorder should not begin until articulation is assessed fully in terms of the number of consonant phonemes produced correctly and the number of consonant phonemes produced incorrectly. The consistency of these errors needs to be noted as well as the phonetic contexts in which production is both correct and incorrect.

The writer proposes that all consonants be tested according to their functions in speech of either releasing or arresting the syllable. When an articulation error is found, the error needs to be described in terms of its function and in terms of type, omission, distortion, and substitution.

The two articulation evaluation forms shown allow for relatively easy notation of phonemic errors according to consistency and the two dimensions of consonant function and type. Stimulus words are not presented, leaving the examiner the freedom to supply the words deemed necessary for initial testing of the error phoneme. The words can be chosen as needed from the materials included in this book. Two words only are used for a consonant sound during the initial test, one word to release the consonant and another to arrest it. Additional words are introduced during subsequent

Consonant Articulation Evaluation
Consonants as Singles

Phoneme	Arrest				Release			
	Stimulus Word	Omis.	Dist.	Sub.	Stimulus Word	Omis.	Dist.	Sub.
m								
n								
ŋ						2	2	2
p								
b								
t								
d								
k								
g								
h		1	1	1				
w		1	1					
j		1	1	1				
r		1	1	1				
l								
f								
v								
θ								
ð								
s								
z								
ʃ								
ʒ						3	3	3
tʃ								
dʒ								

Number
  of errors

1. Sound does not function to arrest syllable in isolated word.
2. Sound does not function to release syllable in isolated word.
3. Sound does not function to release initial syllable in isolated word.

Vocalic [r] and Vocalic [l] Assessment

Phoneme	Initial				Medial				Final			
	Stimulus Word	Omis.	Dist.	Sub.	Stimulus Word	Omis.	Dist.	Sub.	Stimulus Word	Omis.	Dist.	Sub
ɝ												
ɚ					4	4	4					
l̩					4	4	4					

Number
of errors

4. Sound does not appear in initial position in isolated word.

testing to further evaluate the consistency and ease of correctability of the error. The principal two-element blends involving /s/, /r/, /l/, and /w/ may also be tested. Other blends are not included because they are too numerous (over 150) and appear relatively infrequently. The drill material in the book includes many other blends for further speech testing if indicated or for speech drills. The test order follows the arrangement of the drill material in the book, with nasals appearing first, followed by the plosives, glides, fricatives, and affricates in that order. Semivowel [l] and consonant glide [r] are included with the consonants. However, vocalic [l] and the two vocalic [r]'s appear separately.

The two picture articulation tests previously cited, the Developmental Articulation Test and the Templin-Darley Tests (1960) can be used for the nonreader with the form included here. Clinicians can develop their own picture tests, whether an entirely different instrument from the two cited, or a derivative developed by adding new words to these tests when further testing is indicated for a particular sound or if a particular picture seems unsuitable. Actual testing time using pictures can be made relatively short through the use of pictures which designate nouns only. The child is directed to name the pictures presented to him. The following kind of simple directions can be given quickly before beginning the test:

I am going to show you many interesting pictures of things that you will like; tell me their names. If you don't know the name for the picture, ask me the name and I'll tell you. If you get tired or want to stop for any reason, let me know and we'll take a break. But we won't stop too much because there are a lot of pictures here and I would like to show them all to you.

Consonant Articulation Evaluation

Consonants in Two-Element Blends

(Mark Element Incorrect in Blend)

Stimulus Word or Words	s	r	l	w	Omis.	Dist.	Sub.
	sm						
	sn						
	sp						
	sp₅						
		pr	pl				
		br	bl				
	st						
	st₅						
		tr		tw			
		dr		dw			
	sk	kr	kl	kw			
	sk₅	gr	gl				
	sw	fr	fl				
		ɵr					

Number of errors

Consonants in Three-Element Blends

	skr						
	str						
	skw						
	spl						
	spr						

Number of errors

5. Two-element blends arrest and release syllable; all other two-element blends release syllable only.

The child will usually name each picture following these instructions, stopping only when he does not know the name. The child imitates the name if he does not already know it. Templin (1947) found that results were similar whether the child named spontaneously or imitated. She concluded that the best method for eliciting verbal responses to pictures should be "adapted to the needs of a specific child." The child should feel comfortable and not threatened by the test, the examiner, or the procedure. If he feels frightened or insecure, it is best to stop for a while and attempt to develop feelings of security. Test results will be invalid if psychological reactions interfere with verbal responses.

While administering the test, the examiner might occasionally interject the question "What is this?" before presenting a picture in order to relieve the monotony. Frequent smiles, laughter, and nods or indications of approval by the examiner will relieve any monotony and motivate the child to continue naming until completion of the test.

The goal of evaluating the articulation of the child should be kept in mind throughout the test. The child's articulation can be assessed with slight difficulty if he continues to name without interruptions or questioning by the examiner. Too many questions or verbal remarks by the examiner prolong the test unduly, reducing the motivation of the child and his emotional involvement in the procedure. If the child is naming, the inherent rhythm of the test developed by his continuation of naming will maintain the verbal behavior of naming until the test is completed. However, interjections and remarks by the examiner can interfere with the test and disturb any rhythm pattern established by the child.

The child's spontaneous speaking should be assessed prior to the start of the test and following completion of the test. Informal discussion of topics which are of interest to the child will stimulate the child to speak: the child's family, favorite sport, favorite school subject, favorite season of the year, favorite sport, etc. A child who produces a particular sound incorrectly during the testing will usually produce the sound correctly in some phonetic context during spontaneous conversation, either as a single or in blends. Careful listening to the child, and sufficient sampling of the child's speech, will usually uncover a word or words in which production is correct. Notation should be made of these words. These words, of course, will furnish material for initial therapy sessions. The author tested and conversed with a youngster for an hour, finding no words containing correct production of the /s/ or /z/ phonemes. The error was described as consistent. When the child enquired about his *sister*, however, the /s/ releasing the initial syllable was produced correctly. Using this word as a starting point, the child was able to produce this sound correctly in the words *sit* and *sip*, which involve similar phonetic contexts, during a thirty minute lesson the following day.

When an error is consistent in all test words and spontaneous speech, integral or multiple sensory stimulation may provide phonetic environments in which correct production results (Milisen, 1954). Integral stimulation begins with the clinician's production of the sound in words. The child hears the sound, sees placements of the sound and articulators involved,

Integral Stimulation

Consonants as Singles

	Arrest				Release				Non-sense Syl-lable			
Pho-neme	Stim-ulus Word	Impr.	Unch.	Cor.	Stim-ulus Word	Impr.	Unch.	Cor.		Impr.	Unch.	Cor.
m												
n												
ŋ					2	2	2	2				
p												
b												
t												
d												
k												
g												
h	1	1	1	1								
w	1	1	1	1								
j	1	1	1	1								
r	1	1	1	1								
l												
f												
v												
θ												
ð												
s												
z												
ʃ					3	3	3	3				
ʒ												
tʃ												
dʒ												

1. Sound does not function to arrest syllable in isolated word.
2. Sound does not function to release syllable in isolated word.
3. Sound does not function to release initial syllable in isolated word.

Vocalic [r] and Vocalic [l]

	Initial				Medial				Final			
Pho-neme	Stim-ulus Word	Impr.	Unch.	Cor.	Stim-ulus Word	Impr.	Unch.	Cor.	Stim-ulus Word	Impr.	Unch.	Cor.
ɝ												
ɚ	4	4	4	4								
l̩	4	4	4	4								

4. Sound does not appear in initial position in isolated word.

Integral Stimulation

Consonants in Two- and Three-Element Blends

Stimulus Word or Words	s	r	l	w	Unch.	Impr.	Cor.
sm							
sn							
sp							
sp₅	pr	pl					
	br	bl					
st							
st₅							
	tr		tw				
sw	dr		dw				
sk	kr		kw				
	gr	gl					
sk₅							
	fr	fl					
	θr						
skr							
str							
skw							
spl							
spr							

5. Two-element blends arrest and release syllable; all other two-element blends release syllable only.

and feels oral pressure as the sound is released. The child repeats the words following several presentations by the examiner. Comparison is made of production by the examiner and that of the child. If the error persists with the initial word, the examiner presents the word again or presents a different word. The child repeats as before. If the error persists in phonetic contexts in words containing the consonant as a single phoneme, the procedure is repeated with words in which the consonant functions as an element in a blend. If the error persists in blends as well as in singles, the procedure should be repeated with the sound in nonsense syllables and in "isolation," with the recognition that no consonant can function in isolation, as the release of the consonant takes place only with the assistance of a neutral vowel (Stetson, 1951). If correct production occurs with words, integral stimulation is not necessary for the sound in nonsense syllables. However, if correct production does not occur in words, production is tested in nonsense syllables. The error phoneme is tested as it arrests or releases nonsense syllables involving a variety of phonetic contexts. The test forms shown allow for notation of correct, improved, or unchanged production of the phoneme in words and nonsense syllables following integral stimulation. The McDonald Deep Test can be very useful in exploration of phonetic environments in which consonant production may be correct. However, the aim is to find words in which production is correct as quickly as possible. Thus as soon as an effective nonsense syllable combination is found, words which contain this phonetic context and related phonetic contexts are quickly utilized in therapy.

The tasks of arresting and releasing a consonant are usually easiest in one-syllable words which have only one phoneme in addition to the error consonant. Attention can be directed almost entirely to the function of the consonant. The arresting function seems to be easier for older children than the releasing function. The breath has been started already, and apparently the consonant function can be superimposed on the breath stream more easily than it can start the breath stream. Younger children have more difficulties arresting the breath stream than releasing it. Apparently the child beginning to talk is more aware of sounds which begin words than of sounds which end words. He develops sounds in the final position after they are included in the initial position. Further mention will be made of this observation later. Testing for articulation should pay attention to words in which the articulation tasks are presumably easiest and in which, therefore, articulation might be superior.

If production is not correct in either words or nonsense syllables following integral stimulation, notation should be made as to whether production has been improved. A sound will be corrected easiest in the environment in which consonant production is the most nearly correct. Very few children show no improvement of production in words or nonsense syllables following stimulation. The author has had very few children who could not start at least at the nonsense syllable level in therapy; most children start immediately at the word level. If the error persists, however, without improvement following stimulation, there is justification for beginning speech therapy at the earliest level of auditory discrimination at which the child can be taught to recognize and identify correct production. Even here, however, the child should be allowed to produce the sound as quickly as possible in words, both for the motivation of the child and to hasten the articulation learning process.

As examples of the use of integral stimulation, the author has seen children who produce the /s/ incorrectly in all phonetic contexts during the initial articulation test. During integral stimulation, one child produced the sound incorrectly in the words *see, saw,* and *toss.* However, the sound was produced correctly in the words *bus* and *mess.* Apparently lip closure for the labials /b/ and /m/ did not allow for tongue protrusion and distortion. Another child produced the sound correctly in some one-syllable words but not in *toss* or the two-syllable *basement*. The tongue elevation for /t/ in *toss* carried over to other sounds, causing the /s/ error. The distortion in *basement* suggested that the length of the word had an adverse influence on phonemic production. Children have been seen who produce the /f/ correctly in the words *off* and *if* but who distort the sound in the words *fist* and *elephant*. Word length and lingual elevation apparently contribute to the inconsistent distortion of the /f/, as with the /s/.

A child with consistent distortions of /k/ was observed to produce the phoneme correctly in the one word *key*. Obviously word length was responsible for the errors. Therapy started with the word *key* and gradually involved lengthier words. The writer has encountered numerous children who distorted the /ʃ/ but who could produce the phoneme correctly during integral stimulation when either releasing or arresting a syllable with only one other sound. The words *she, shoe,* and *ash* may be handled with success by these children, or any nonsense syllable combining the /ʃ/ with a vowel may be tried.

Frequently articulation is acceptable in isolated words, but errors appear in connected speech. This becomes apparent in comparing articulation during the formal test with articulation during spontaneous speech. Obviously blending of sounds, rate, stress, and grammatical dimensions contribute to this kind of inconsistency and need to be considered during therapy.

Therapy can begin following the assessment, using for the initial lessons the words in which the sound is produced correctly. Speech therapy results will be quickest generally with the sounds which are the most inconsistent. An error phoneme involving the /t/ which is produced correctly in /st/ blends and to release a syllable will be corrected more easily than the /s/ which is produced correctly in blends only. But the /s/ probably will be corrected more easily than the /k/ if no word or phonetic context has been found in which production of /k/ is correct. Among sounds which are produced incorrectly in all test words, the ones corrected most easily will be those which are produced correctly in more words following integral stimulation. When sounds are equally inconsistent, some consideration should be given to the order of mastery of consonants by the child without articulation difficulty, with nasals, plosives, glides, fricatives, and affricates in that order. Visibility of phoneme should be a consideration also, so that in considering plosives the easily seen /p/ and /b/ would be handled before the /k/ and /g/, which are not visible. For fricatives, /f/, /v/, /θ/, and /ð/ can be seen more easily than others. Among the fricatives, the ones requiring finer lingual adjustments and thus more complicated alteration of the breath stream, will be more difficult to correct than the labiodental or interdentals, which are easily seen. The /f/, /v/, /θ/, /ð/ can probably be corrected more easily than the /ʃ/ and /s/. The frequency of the sound in the language should receive some consideration in the selection of the sound for training. An error in production of a frequently appearing phoneme will obviously have a greater effect on speech intelligibility than an error in a sound which does not appear very frequently in the language. But this factor alone appears to be of less importance clinically than consistency of the error and age of mastery by normal-speaking children. Feelings of success are greater motivating forces than other factors in articulation training. The tasks chosen first should be those which offer the greatest possibility for success.

When the child produces the sound correctly in a word, he should be made aware of the correctness of production. As other words are used in which the sound is produced incorrectly, he should be made aware of the incorrectness of the production. The "do" language is stressed, a concept which has been found very meaningful in stuttering therapy (Williams, 1957; Johnson et al., 1967). The manner of production in which the sound is correct is contrasted with the manner of production in which the sound is incorrect. For example, the /s/ may be produced correctly in blends but the tongue may be placed interdentally when the sound functions as a single consonant to arrest or release a syllable. As the youngster compares the two manners of production, he becomes aware that the sound is produced correctly when the tongue is contained within the mouth but that it is distorted when the tongue is placed outside of the mouth. A blending of the auditory, kinesthetic, and tactual modalities is used immediately. The auditory modality passes final judgment on the correctness of production. The other modalities assist in production, with kinesthetic arousal for placements which are correct and incorrect as the auditory modality perceives production to be either correct or incorrect. When correct production is heard, the child will learn to attend to what he does. When incorrect production is heard, he will also learn to attend to what he does. As the frequencies of correct production increase, he will begin to favor the manner of production and the breath stream alterations which result in correct production. Consequently he will begin to use the breath stream alterations which result in incorrect production less and less.

ARTICULATION TREATMENT AND THE WHOLE WORD METHOD

The use of the whole word method in therapy has as its premise the rewarding of correct responses. Incorrect responses are corrected as a result of comparing the two different productions. The child compares himself with himself, in a manner of speaking. The clinician needs to be very aware of the factors affecting the production and needs to relate this awareness to the child. For example, children frequently distort the /f/ if the tongue is involved in the production. One particular child had many correct productions of the phoneme and also many productions which were incorrect. Dialogue and communication were very effective in working with this child. This child was given the following meaningful explanations: "Remember, this sound is made with the upper teeth over the lower lip. If you involve your tongue, you produce a sound which is not correct. You just produced the sound correctly in the two words *off* and *if*, but the tongue made the sound incorrect in *fit*."

Abundant praise should be used, stressing reward. Responses should be sought which can be rewarded. A cleft palate youngster was apparently discouraged by slow progress. To overcome this, we started each lesson by reviewing the sounds which were "perfect." Then we considered the sounds which were almost "perfect," in which definite phonetic contexts yielded the errors. Finally, we considered the few remaining sounds which were "less than almost perfect." We could discuss and rejoice over the sounds produced correctly and vow to produce all sounds correctly.

Recognizing allophonic variations in the speech of children with articulation errors, the two dimensions of the problem need to be explored fully with each individual child, the one instance in which consonant production is correct and the other instance in which consonant production is incorrect. The phenomenon of inconsistency of error production or the dimension of correctness-incorrectness can be related to the following factors: (1) consonant function, (2) voicing, (3) length of word, (4) vowel shaping, (5) blend production, (6) placement, (7) stress, and (8) rate. The drill materials in this book consider the effects of the first six variables in speech assessment and therapy with the child. The effect of the last two variables, stress and rate, on articulation can be handled through extending the length of the speech utterance beyond the single-word level, as has been detailed in a previous section.

Each of the variables will be explained in detail. Examples will be given freely from the author's experiences with children with whom therapy time was shortened considerably through the exploration and utilization of these variables.

CONSONANT FUNCTION

Frequently a child may be able to produce a sound correctly in some words when the consonant releases the syllable. Conversely, another child may produce the sound correctly only in order to arrest the syllable. As an example of the first instance, the author has worked with children who correctly produce the /p/ in the one syllable words *pay*, *pie*, and *pig* but omit the sound when it releases syllables beyond the first syllable or when it arrests the syllable. Correction of the error can begin by drilling first on more one-syllable words in which the phoneme releases the syllable until the sound is produced correctly in releasing all one-syllable words. Each noun is then prefaced by the function words *my, the,* and *a*. From the units *a pie, the pie, my pie,* the children proceed to *apple, supper,* and *carpet* and other bisyllable words with the words divided into separate syllables enabling the children to recognize that the /p/ functions to release the second syllable of the words. Word list drills follow, with gradual mastery of the phoneme to release the syllable in all phonetic contexts. The arresting function of the plosive can be taught through subtle handling of the drill material in which the phoneme releases the syllable. From the word *apple,* which has been involved in drill on the /p/ as the releasing element, the child stops momentarily following release of the first syllable as he occludes the lips and relaxes them, resulting in the syllable /æp/. Words are formed quickly with this syllable: *cap, nap, sap, lap, map,* and *wrap*. The word *carpet* previously introduced is divided into the two words *car* and *pet*. The words are spoken together pausing after release of the /p/ without producing the other sounds in the word *pet*. The word *carp* results from this. The words *harp, sharp,* and *warp* are introduced immediately.

Preschool and early elementary schoolchildren omit final phonemes very frequently and will learn quite easily to produce the sound correctly in drill words. The child needs to be made aware, however, that not all words end with consonants, that many words end with vowels. The child may generalize production to other words which are arrested by other consonants. As examples, a child successfully produced /p/ to arrest the words *cap* and *cup*. She referred to her pet as a *cap* (*cat*) and to her *cup* (*cut*) from a knife. Later when work was begun with /m/ to arrest syllables, she talked about *seeming* (*seeing*) her friend. She asked me, "Do you *knom* (*know*) my teacher?"

The author has worked with children who produced the /p/ correctly to arrest the syllable but who were generally unable to produce the sound correctly to release the syllables. The children were taught to release the syllable with /p/ through systematic extension of drill material containing words in which /p/ acts as an arresting element in this manner: As the noun is combined with other words, the function of the consonant can change from that of an arresting element to that of a releasing element if the word following the noun begins with a vowel. For example, by inserting the words *cup, cap, top,* and *rope* in the phrases "*The* (*cup*) (*top*) (*cap*) (*rope*) *is mine*," "*The* (*cup*) (*etc.*) *is yours*," "*The* (*cup*) (*etc.*) *in your hand*," "*The* (*cup*) (*etc.*) *it was lost*," the /p/, while functioning as an arresting element with these words in isolation, becomes a releasing element by blending with the words *is, in, it* in the newly formed words *cupiz, topiz, cupin, topin, cupit,* and *topit.* By isolating the "new words" *cupiz, cupin, cupit,* etc., drill centers immediately on /p/ as a releasing element. By dividing the unit into syllables and stopping the breath pulse just before release, /p/ functions in this context as an unaspirated plosive. If the /p/ is released following the pause, it becomes a releasing element. From drilling on half a unit, so to speak, the task of releasing the syllable now becomes possible, as the lips which have been occluded to stop the pulse are now opened to release the syllable. The words *pit, pin, pill, pig,* etc., may be produced correctly now because of their similarity to the syllables in the phrases. More complicated phonetic contexts are presented until production of /p/ is correct consistently.

The author has worked with youngsters from the second and third grades who had errors with the production of the plosives /k/ and /g/. Careful listening and testing revealed that the sound was produced correctly to arrest the one-syllable words *book, lock,* and *rock.* However, the /t/ phoneme was produced for the sound in words in which the /k/ functioned as a releasing element. At the initial meetings, the children learned to produce the /k/ correctly as the arresting element in more one-syllable words. Nouns were paired and joined by the connective *and* to form the phrases *book and sock, lock and rock.* As a result of blending the noun with the connective, the arresting elements in the word *book* in the first phrase and the word *lock* in the second phrase functioned as releasing elements for *and* in both phrases. In essence, the syllable /kɛ/ was produced as the noun word and connective were blended. For drill purposes, two syllables were isolated from the phrase and the following phonetic sequences were repeated numerous times: /bʊ-kɛ-kɛ-kɛ/, /rɑ-kɛ-kɛ-kɛ/, /sɑ-kɛ-kɛ-kɛ/, etc. We were now able to isolate the nonsense syllable [kɛ], resulting in correct production of the /k/ in the isolated syllable. The syllable was arrested by the consonants /n/ and /pt/ to form the words *Ken* (the name of the brother of one youngster), and *kept.* Next the schwa or neutral vowel /ʌ/ was combined with the phoneme to form the syllable /kʌ/, and the child was able to produce the sound correctly in this syllable. This syllable was arrested by the consonants /p/, /b/, /m/, /f/, /t/, and /d/ to form the words *cup, cub, come, cuff, cut,* and *cud.* The /k/ was introduced next as a releasing element in the syllable /ko/, and the syllable was arrested by the consonants /m/, /tʃ/, /l/, /t/, and /d/ to form the words *comb, coach, coal, coat,* and *code.* The words formed from the three syllables /kʌ/, /kɛ/, and /ko/ were combined together for more extensive word drill. Longer speech units were developed by prefacing nouns with function words and verbs with pronouns. Finally, the children drilled on all the /k/ words contained in this book, reading words when they were able, and repeating words they were not able to read. Pictures were secured for words which the children were not able to read and for nonreaders. Inconsistent errors involving consonants to release the syllable can be handled through utilization of the morpheme /ɪz/ with nouns and verbs, which pluralizes the nouns but is used for singular verbs. For example, the /tʃ/ arrests the syllabic nouns and verbs *catch, match,* and *hatch* but releases the second syllable in the words *catches, matches,* and *watches.* Correction can occur rather quickly by strongly releasing the affricate and then quickly blending the morpheme with it. From *catches,* other words can include *catching, ketchup,* and *kachoo.*

The functions of the consonant in releasing and arresting the breath stream need to be explored particularly with children having an organic or structural basis for the articulation disorder. The consonant functioning to release the syllable requires more breath pressure than the consonant which arrests the syllable (Black, 1950). Children with organic difficulties have particular difficulty in the development of oral breath pressure, and therefore they can be expected to handle the arresting consonant easier than the releasing consonant. Considerable investigation has pointed to the inadequacy of breath pressure with cleft palate speakers (Spriestersbach and Powers, 1959; Spriestersbach et al., 1961). The writer has worked with several cleft palate children who had learned to produce acceptable /ʃ/ and /s/ to arrest the syllable, but who experienced considerable trouble in producing the sound to release the syllable. However, as explained previously, through involving drill words in more phonetic contexts involving longer utterances, the function of the consonant changed from arresting the syllable to releasing it. For example, the fricative /ʃ/ was produced by several children correctly in the word *wash.* A two-word utterance was developed by prefacing the word with the pronouns *I, you,* and *we,* with the sound still functioning to arrest the syllable at the completion of the phrase. Extended utterances were developed by adding words which begin with vowels to the two-word phrase: *I wash eggs, I wash apples, I wash animals, I wash alligators, I wash anything, I wash up.* As the child spoke these phrases, he was directed not to pause after the word *wash* but to say immediately the words which complete the phrase. In essence, the /ʃ/ functions with all of these phrases to release the initial syllables of the words following the word *wash.*

These examples illustrate that the task of correcting consonant function inconsistency can be easier with fricatives than plosives, for fricatives are continuants and therefore can be sustained. When a fricative is produced correctly as an arresting element, the child needs only to sustain the fricative to have the sound in "isolation." When the fricative can be produced as a releasing element, it can be isolated, identified, and then quickly combined with vowels to function as an arresting element.

As further examples, the child may be able to produce the /f/ correctly in the words *if, off*, and *life*, but incorrectly in releasing syllables. Through addition of syntactically appropriate words which begin with vowels, the function of the fricative changes from arresting the syllable to releasing it. Such short phrases as the following may be utilized: *if I can, if I may, if I want; off it, off in a minute; My life is good, Her life is happy, for the life of me.* Discussions may occur, with the clinician pointing out to the child the reasons for the variable productions in the different phonetic contexts. The words *fight, fine, find* can follow after success with the phrases which begin with *if I*. Such words as *fish, fill, fix*, and *fit* can follow after success with the phrases which begin with *off in, off it*, and *my life is*. Other words may be selected of similar phonetic context and with systematic enlargement of the responses.

Words following arresting fricatives which begin with consonants can be considered within the context of the phrases. The resulting phonetic contexts may be more difficult to manage, perhaps even requiring the child to stop the fricative before production of the consonant which follows immediately. McDonald (1964A) discusses the use of contiguous consonants in articulation therapy, not allowing pause time, however.

Plosives are somewhat more difficult to utilize in changing the consonant function because production needs to stop before releasing. The arresting function can be changed to the releasing function rather easily, as has been described in earlier examples. The change from releasing function may offer more difficulty but can usually be done, with therapeutic results occurring much faster than if each function were considered as separate and different.

VOICING

Considerable therapy time can be saved if attention is paid very early to the phenomenon of voicing inconsistency. If the child is able to produce the voiced sound correctly but not the voiceless counterpart, or, vice versa, is able to produce the voiceless sound but not the voiced counterpart, drill material can be prepared to facilitate early mastery of the voiced or voiceless counterpart. The writer was working with a fourth grade youngster who produced the /k/ phoneme correctly to both release and arrest the breath pulse, but who either distorted or omitted the voiced counterpart /g/. Early drills were prepared with contrasting pairs of words which differed only in the one element. The following words were contrasted: *come, gum; came, game; could, good;* etc. The child learned to produce the error sound correctly in the paired words through the use of the auditory modality alone. If a child has difficulty correcting the error through listening alone, placement of his fingers over the thyroid notch or Adam's apple of the clinician will enable the child to feel the vibrations for the voiced sounds, and absence of vibration will be noted with voiceless sounds. A child can duplicate the vibration or lack of it easily when he feels his own Adam's apple.

Longer speech units were selected which favor quick learning of the voiced sound. The missing word in the phrase unit "*The* _____ *is mine*" was filled in with nouns of one syllable which were arrested by the /k/ phoneme. As the words *book, rock, sock*, etc., are produced in the phrase, the /k/ tends to become a voiced element because of its location between two voiced elements.

The author achieved success with several youngsters who were not producing the /d/ phoneme correctly in words but who produced the voiceless counterpart /t/ correctly. As with the previous example, contrasting pairs of words were drilled on which differed only with the one element. The /t/ words were inserted in the sentence "*The* (*hat*) (*coat*) (*rat*) *is mine.*" The /t/ phoneme approaches a /d/ in the phrase because of its location between two voiced sounds. Joining nouns together by use of the connective *and* sets up a phonetic environment in which the voiceless consonant tends to become voiced.

LENGTH OF WORD

Children frequently will be able to produce a sound correctly in one-syllable words but will distort or omit the sound in a longer word.* Drill on the shorter words in which sound production is already correct with stress on the problem phoneme intensifies auditory discrimination, enabling the child to attend better to correct production of the sound. The process of correctly producing the sound in longer words is possible after the child has attended to correct production in the shorter words. Division of the longer words into syllabic components will be of great help because the syllabication in essence reduces the longer word into shorter words. The semivowel [l], for example, may be produced correctly in such one-syllable words as *lie* and *lay* by attending to tongue elevation and lip spreading. If the lips become rounded in the speaking of these words, /w/ is likely to be produced as the releasing element. The error can be corrected in these words by unrounding the lips. The one-syllable words *lie* and *lay* can now

---

* The so-called medial classification of a sound is possible only with longer words. One-syllable words have only initial and final consonants, the former releasing the syllables and the latter arresting them.

become bisyllabic in *lying* and *later*, and polysyllabic in the phrases *lying is* and *later on*. The consonant glide [r] as we shall see in a separate section, may be produced correctly in the words *row* and *run* but be distorted in the longer word *arrow* or phrase *I run*. The lingual adjustments for correct production of the fricatives /ʃ/, /s/, and /z/ are easily learned with one-syllable words but become increasingly difficult with longer words. Placement of the upper teeth over the lower lip for production of /f/ and /v/ is readily learned with short words, but the placement becomes more difficult with lengthier words. Children with inconsistent articulation errors will be more likely to produce the sound correctly in short one-syllable words than in words which contain more than one syllable. However, the phenomenon of inconsistency suggests that this kind of articulation behavior is not always true, for some children will produce the sound correctly in longer words and incorrectly in shorter words. A child with multiple articulation errors may produce one sound correctly in some words exceeding one syllable but incorrectly in words of only one syllable, and yet the reverse may be true for another sound, with correct production in one-syllable words only. Careful listening to the speech of the child while he produces the sound in a number of different phonetic contexts will provide the information necessary to decide on the relationship between word length and the consistency of the error.

VOWEL SHAPING

Consonant production will be affected by the contiguous vowel sounds. The writer has worked with numerous youngsters who distorted the fricative /s/ and /ʃ/ when they were followed by back vowels requiring rounding of lips. Production of the phonemes was correct when followed by front vowels requiring lip spreading. As the lips were rounded, the tongue placement tended to shift from contact with the alveolar ridge to interdental contact. As children learned to retain the lingual placement against the alveolar ridge with rounded or spread lips, they learn to produce the /s/ correctly in all phonetic contexts. Conversely, there have been children who substituted the /θ/ for the /s/ when the sound was followed by front vowels but for whom production was correct in the phonetic context involving back vowels. As a general rule, the tongue is encouraged more toward interdental tongue placement with front vowels than with back vowels. The author has worked with children who distorted the consonant [r] when it preceded a back lip rounding vowel but who correctly produce the sound when it preceded front vowels. As with therapy for the /s/ distorted under similar circumstances, the lingual placement found with the front vowels had to be retained with the back vowels.

Movement of the rear portion of the tongue can also explain inconsistent articulation errors involving consonant phonemes. The author has worked with children who correctly produced the /g/ and /k/ phonemes only when the sounds were associated with the back vowels /o/ and /u/. By drilling on the words *coat*, *cold*, *cool*, *goat*, *gold*, and *goose*, the children learned to listen to and "feel" the correct production of the /k/ and /g/ in the words. We then isolated the /ku/, and /gu/, /ko/ and /go/ units from the words. Words were constructed with the /k/ and /g/ in combination with other vowels. General drill on the /k/ and /g/ phonemes followed.

The size of the mouth opening which effects vowel production may also hinder correct production of consonant sounds, since the tongue may not have sufficient room to elevate and contact the alveolar ridge or soft palate. Production of the phonemes /t/, /d/, /n/, and /l/ may be affected by too small a mouth opening. In rare instances, the size of the mouth opening may even be too large for the child, thus making it impossible for the tongue to contact the palate. A word of caution needs to be sounded in working with this problem, because while articulation production might be assisted by reducing the size of mouth opening, voice quality might become aberrant. The writer has worked with cleft palate children who mastered correct production of the /l/ phoneme by reducing the size of the mouth opening only to find that the reduced mouth opening intensified the degree of hypernasality. Further therapy was necessary in order to reduce the hypernasality. As in all things, a wise perspective needs to be established in articulation therapy, with careful attention to the effect of articulation improvement on other aspects of speech.

BLEND PRODUCTION

Inconsistent articulation errors are particularly prominent with the /l/, /r/, and /s/ phonemes. As mentioned numerous times previously, sounds may be produced correctly when part of a blend. The reverse situation may also occur: sounds may be produced correctly as single sounds but may be produced incorrectly as elements of blends. Lingual adjustments are often the factor responsible for the inconsistency. For example, the /s/ may be produced correctly in the /st/ and /sl/ blends. As the tongue is elevated for production of the /l/ and /t/, the movement is so quick that interdental tongue placement and resulting distortion of the /s/ phoneme is not possible such as would occur with production of the /s/ phoneme as a single consonant. Frequently utilization of the blends /sm/ and /sp/ will help correct distortion of /s/ if the distortion occurs because of interdental tongue placement. The /m/ and /p/ phonemes require lip occlusion, and thus the child may be prevented from protruding his tongue for production of the /s/ if he anticipates production of the labial sounds. Awareness of /s/ placement for the blends and stopping of the blends before the second element is produced can usually result in learning of placements which are correct and incorrect for production of the sound.

If the error occurs in the /s/ blends as the tongue is elevated for production of the /t/ and /l/ but production is correct for the /s/ as a single element, blends need to be divided into the separate sounds which the child hears himself produce correctly. Correct blend production can occur as the separate sounds are slowly and carefully joined together to form again the blend. Frequently the velar plosives /k/ and /g/ are produced correctly when associated with the /r/ in blends. As with the /s/, the blend needs to be divided into the separate sounds with ear training for the sounds as parts of blends and then for the sounds as separate phonemes. The semivowel [l] distortion because of lip rounding may not occur in blends. To drill on lip rounding as an isolated event may introduce an artificial component which does not occur if lip rounding occurs naturally in production of blends.

Discussion of therapy involving /r/ blends will be discussed in a later section.

PLACEMENT

Because of psychological and physiological differences between speakers and the abilities of some persons to compensate for structural limitations, as was mentioned earlier, descriptions cannot be made of exact and precise placements for productions of consonants. However, general statements may be made concerning minimal placement requirements. For example, the bilabial plosives cannot be produced correctly unless the lips are occluded. The fricative /s/ cannot be produced correctly unless the tongue placement allows the air stream to pass between it and a cutting edge. If minimal placement requirements are not met, however, distortions occur, and yet if the distortions are inconsistent minimal placement requirements must be met in other phonetic contexts. I have worked with children who distorted the /p/ in releasing syllables because their lips were separated. Production was correct in arresting the syllable because lips were occluded. The /s/ and /ʃ/ fricatives are distorted if the teeth are separated thus not allowing the air stream to pass over a cutting edge. Children are likely to produce the /s/ correctly if the /s/ phoneme is an element in the /sm/ blend because the /m/ requires lip closure which may result in dental occlusion thus in proper production of /s/. Even when blends are not used, the fricatives are produced correctly when the teeth are occluded and produced incorrectly if the teeth are separated. Phonetic contexts can usually be found in which productions are correct and incorrect because of these dental relationships.

Production of the affricates /dʒ/ and /tʒ/ may result in similar variable distortions. For correct production of these sounds, the breath stream must first be stopped by the teeth as the uppers and lowers meet, usually in midline, and then must be released through an open oral cavity. Distortions result if the breath stream is not stopped or if stoppage occurs without properly involving the upper and lower teeth. If the child has an overbite, class II malocclusion, correct production of the fricatives in all phonetic contexts is probably not possible unless orthodontic treatment is done. In the event of severe malocclusions and open bite, speech therapy for fricative errors should probably not begin until orthodontic treatment is instituted.

Lingual placement is responsible for many consonant errors. The consonants which require tongue-tip elevation are /t/, /d/, /n/, and /l/ and are four of the six consonants which appear most frequently in large samples of speech (Fairbanks, 1960). Children may elevate the tongue for correct production of one or more of the tongue-tip sounds but may either keep the tongue flat or place it interdentally for other tongue-tip sounds, thus distorting them. Yet if the tongue can be elevated to produce one of the sounds correctly in words, it can be elevated to produce the other sounds also. Contrasting word lists can be utilized which differ only with the specific tongue-tip sound. Words in which the sound is produced correctly can be contrasted with the words in which the sound is produced incorrectly. For example, if these sounds are produced correctly with the exception of a distortion of the semivowel [l], one-syllable words with the plosives can illustrate that the breath stream is stopped for the plosive by tight placement of the tongue tip against the alveolar ridge, but that for production of the [l] the tongue tip is placed loosely against the ridge with the breath stream passing without interruption over the sides of the tongue. Occasionally phonemic production is correct for [l] but distorted for the other tongue tip sounds because of interdental tongue placement. The plosives /t/ and /d/ may become distorted fricatives because the breath stream is not stopped, as would occur if the tongue contacted the alveolar ridge. The placement for production of these sounds and the concepts of tightness and looseness of tongue placement will become apparent as a result of correct production without the need for excessive verbal description, phonetic diagrams, or mirror observation, these three latter methods being used quite extensively by many clinicians. If the sound can be produced correctly and with ease by contrasting in the manner described, the techniques of diagramming and mirror observation become unnecessary, time consuming, and may well prove to be tedious as well as unmotivating to many children. Further, these techniques can slow therapeutic results considerably.

A chief error in the speech of young children, substitution of /t/ for /k/, is frequently accounted for by tongue-tip elevation to contact the alveolar ridge for production of /k/. The error can be corrected almost at once by cautioning the child against moving the tongue tip, and requiring him to move the rear portion of the tongue instead, when producing /k/.

Occasionally all tongue-tip sounds may be produced incorrectly because of limited tongue elevation. These children do all of their speaking without involving any area above the upper teeth. They frequently swallow all foods and liquids by thrusting their tongues interdentally or against the upper teeth. The thrust of the tongue against the teeth can cause malocclusions. Orthodontic intervention is not always successful until tongue-tip placement is changed during swallowing from contacting the teeth to that of contacting the alveolar ridge or environs. Tongue thrust during swallowing in this latter area will do no harm because bone cannot be affected by the tight seal which is required before swallowing can be completed. As therapy is done for correction of the consonants, tongue placement during swallowing can be handled as well. The author has described elsewhere the role of the speech pathologist in the area of tongue thrusting and procedures which could remedy the faulty tongue placement, which leads to poor speech and malocclusions (Goda, 1968).

STRESS

Children may have acceptable articulation in short words and phrases. However, articulation errors occur when speech output is extended. Plosives may be distorted because their release is too weak. Fricatives may be muted because of lack of intensity. Articulation can improve as we involve different stress patterns with aspects of duration, pitch, and intensity, the elements associated with stress (Fairbanks, 1960). Initially each element needs to be handled separately, and the single element alone might improve the other two elements and articulation as well. For example, lack of loudness alone may be responsible for faulty pitch and articulation errors. As intensity is increased through development of more adequate breath supply and breath control, articulation also improves because of greater oral breath pressure being available for production of individual consonant sounds.

RATE

Too slow a rate or too rapid a rate may contribute to inconsistent articulation errors. With slow rate articulation may be very labored, whereas with very fast rate articulation may be too rapid to allow sufficient time for correct production of all necessary consonant phonemes in utterances. Some sounds are more distorted than others as a result of faulty rate, and as the rate begins to improve so also will the articulation. Children with organic etiology frequently have severe articulation errors because the rate of speech is too slow and labored. As rate increases, articulation improves, along with stress patterns. The over-all result is greater intelligibility.

However, rate does not always play a significant part with the child who has functional errors. This point needs to be stressed, because parents will frequently state that the child's speech improves if he slows down. The parent believes the child improves because he can be understood better when she directs him to speak slower. However, he is usually repeating the statement and the parent is listening for the second time. Further, the child may speak fewer words in repeating, thus reducing the number of words which need to be understood. Since he is speaking fewer words and these words at a slower rate, the listener will be able to supply missing consonants in words. However, phrasing will usually be faulty. If the child with articulation errors is cautioned to speak slower when there is no rate problem, a more severe speech problem can result.

THERAPY FOR MISARTICULATION OF /r/

A separate section is devoted to therapy for misarticulation of /r/ because of the extreme difficulty children have in mastering production of this sound and the frequency of incorrect production by children with articulation difficulties. Some clinicians prescribe an appliance to control tongue placement for children who misarticulate the /r/ (Garrett, 1968). The inconsistency of the error, the rapidity of tongue movement during running speech, and the impossibility of deciding on the "correct" tongue placement in all phonetic contexts for production of the sound make the utilization of such an appliance highly impractical and unreasonable. Moreover, if an appliance is introduced, speaking is likely to be slow, labored, and unnatural. Correction of /r/ errors will result from appropriate therapeutic methods, as with correction of other consonant errors, without resorting to artificial means.

Clinical observations of children producing the /r/ incorrectly provide evidence that the consonant glide [r] and vocalic [r] are two different sounds, and that a child may have an error with one of the sounds and not the other. Curtis and Hardy (1959) describe three different /r/ sounds, the consonant glide [r], the stressed vocalic [ɝ], and the unstressed vocalic [ɚ]. They discuss the possibility of a fourth /r/, the intervocalic [r], as in such words as *carrot* and *arrow*. However this sound behaves clinically like the consonant glide [r], releasing the second syllable. Errors in these phonetic contexts are related to word length. If the child can produce the glide correctly to release one-syllable words, he needs to learn to release syllables beyond the first in lengthier words.

Children may have errors when they produce one of the /r/ sounds but may produce the other /r/ sounds correctly. Even when there is an error with one of the /r/ sounds, Curtis and Hardy comment on the inconsistency of the error when they provide proof that children "articulate /r/ sounds differently in different phonetic contexts." Careful testing of the speech of children with /r/ misarticulations will reveal the specific /r/ which is defective and the consistency of error.

When evidence is found of the error with the consonant glide only, involvement with the vocalic [r] is not necessary. The error, as with the /s/, needs to be studied as a single sound in various phonetic contexts and as an element in a blend. Production may be correct only in certain blends. For example, Curtis and Hardy report from their sample that correct articulation of the glide consonant [r] was highest for the blends containing stop consonants. Among the stop consonants, correct production was greater with blends containing front-stop consonants than blends containing back-stop consonants. When production of the consonant glide [r] is correct in a blend but not as a single, the blend can be fractionated into the [r] and the additional consonant. Many attempts may need to be carried out before the glide is produced correctly as a single sound. However, if the child is able to produce the sound correctly in the blend, he should eventually be able to produce this sound as a single. When production of the [r] is correct as a single but incorrect in blends, a procedure opposite from the above should be tried. The sounds should be produced first as singles and then blended together. Correction of the glide error occurring only in blends but correct as a single will probably be faster than correction of the error occurring in singles but correct in blends.

Frequently the child misarticulating the /r/ sounds will produce two of the /r/ sounds correctly in some phonetic contexts. These two sounds obviously need to be mastered in more phonetic contexts, and drill on one of the /r/ sounds can be used effectively to master production of the other /r/ sound deviations. The author has worked with youngsters who correctly produced the consonant glide [r] in some blends and the stressed vocalic [ɝ] in a few one-syllable words. Production of the [ɝ], for example, was correct in the words *fur*, *sir*, and *purr*. The time spent on the vocalic element was lengthened. The vowel [ɝ] was produced alone, thus intensifying auditory awareness. The front vowels /i/ and /ɪ/ were isolated and sounded, following production of these words. Gradually the pause time between the words and the vowels was reduced until the words virtually being said were *furry*, *purry*, and *sirry*. After successful production of the [ɝ] in these units, the second syllable in these words was repeated several times. The child was saying /fɝ-ri-ri-ri/ or /fɝ-rɪ-rɪ-rɪ/. From /ri/, success was realized with the words *read*, *real*, *wreathe*, etc. From /rɪ/, success was realized with *rich*, *rim*, *rip*, etc. Bisyllabic words such as *carrot*, *porridge*, *carriage* were introduced with success in the release of the second syllable. Concomitantly the [r] was separated from the blends /br/ and /tr/, in which production was correct. The following words were selected from the child's reader: *bring*, *break*, *bright*, *tree*, *try*, *trick*. The words were produced as a unit, and then the blend was divided into the two elements in the word. The child thus was producing the plosive, pausing, then producing the [r] glide with the rest of the word, and then the word or syllable was spoken several times without the plosive. As an example, the child says *bring, b-ring, ring, ring, ring, brave, b-rave, rave, rave, rave, break, b-reak, reak* (actually, /eɪk, eɪk, eɪk/, etc.). Gradually more and more phonetic contexts were utilized for correction of the sound, until production was essentially correct in all drill words and sentences.

When the error occurs in production of the stressed vocalic [ɝ] but production of the unstressed vocalic [ɚ] is correct, *hammer*, *silver*, *teacher*, and *water* can be contrasted with words which have the stressed vocalic [ɝ]: *early*, *purpose*, *thirteen*, and *thirsty*. The unstressed [ɚ] in the first words in which production is correct is unstressed initially and then stressed with heightened auditory awareness of the acoustic differences between the two /r/'s. Later the words containing the stressed vowels are used in further illustrating the acoustic differences. Words incorporated into short phrases can also be used in correcting one of the vocalic [r]'s if the other is produced correctly. For example, if the error occurs with the unstressed [ɚ], the words *muštárd*, and *effórt* are included in the sentences *The muštárd is mine* and *The effórt is mine*. Stress is reduced gradually until the unstressed [ɚ] is correctly produced. When production is correct with the unstressed vowel but is incorrect with the stressed vowel, the opposite procedure can be tried. The /r/ vowel is unstressed in words in the sentences: *They fuřnísh it* and *They peřmít it*. The proper production occurs as increasing stress is placed gradually on the initial syllables of the words.

It must be understood that the time spent with each phonetic context and separate /r/ sound varies with the individual child. Children who read understand this approach very quickly and thus are usually able to produce words correctly in many phonetic contexts after relatively few lessons, while a child who is a poor or nonreader requires longer periods of time.

Consistent Articulation Errors

While the large majority of articulation errors will be inconsistent, there will occasionally be articulation errors which are consistent and thus produced incorrectly in all phonetic contexts. Careful association of the sound with different vowels will usually reveal a phonetic context in which production of the sound most nearly approximates correct production. This phonetic context furnishes drill material for the initial lessons. As with therapy involving correction of errors produced inconsistently, the child needs to be allowed to see, hear, and feel the production of the phoneme in the nonsense syllable. The different sensory modalities can result in significantly quicker correction of the articulation error than would occur if the stimulus were presented to the auditory modality alone. The child continues to imitate the production of the clinician until the child's production is correct.

When production is correct in the nonsense syllable, words should be introduced as quickly as possible. Many nonsense syllables are themselves one-syllable words. If the particular nonsense syllable is not a word, it should be made into one; the majority of nonsense syllables become words by the addition of a single sound. When the child can produce the sound correctly in a few phonetic contexts, the number of phonetic contexts can by systematically varied until mastery is realized in more phonetic contexts. Then one can utilize materials which are longer than single-word utterances.

To illustrate the procedure with the child whose articulation errors are consistent, the author was working with a second grade youngster who either omitted the /f/ phoneme or substituted the /p/ for it in all phonetic contexts. The child was able to quickly produce the sound in "isolation" by observing, listening to the author's production, and feeling the breath stream as it passed between the upper teeth and lower lip. Involvement of the sound was unsuccessful in all phonetic contexts which required lip rounding or lip spreading. However, production was found to be correct with the /a/ vowel which makes no specific requirement on the lips except that they be separated as the mouth is opened significantly. After numerous repetitions of correct production of the /f/ with the /a/, the sound was involved with the /o/, requiring lip rounding with a relative large mouth opening. Attention was directed to the child's maintaining the same placement with the /f/ blended with the /o/ as he had with the /a/. When the /f/ sound was omitted if combined with either of these vowel sounds, the author would remind the youngster, "You are not doing the same thing now as you did before." Then we would discuss what he was doing differently. The author would describe what he was doing when he produced the sound; the child would report what he saw. Then the child described what he was doing when he produced the sound, and the author described what he saw. The child was then able to combine the /f/ and the /o/ into a syllable. Words were now formed by adding a single sound to the two phonetic combinations /fa/ and /fo/. The words were *far, farm,* and *phone.* Other phonetic environments were introduced, with careful attention to maintenance of the placement as different requirements were made of the lips. Short phrases, as outlined previously, were introduced, serving as a strong motivation to the child who was able to see consistent and rapid progress which immediately involved words. The parents were alert to the improvement and reinforced correct production through praise at home.

4. Further Procedures in Articulation Therapy Adapted to Age Level

This chapter will discuss further procedures to follow and materials to use in speech therapy with persons having articulation disorders. Obviously, the age and personality of the speaker will need to be considered in any therapy program, in addition to the number and consistency of the consonant errors. Persons of all ages, from preschool and school years to adults, can have consonant errors in their speaking. Although the goals of consonant mastery are the same for children and adults, procedures and materials will need to differ with each group.

In order to be maximally effective with all age groups, speech therapy needs to take place in an environment in which there are feelings of trust and respect between the clinician and the defective speaker. Each must feel comfortable and relaxed with the other. In order for speech behavior to change, anxiety has to be minimized as much as possible in all other areas. Although a change is sought in only one element of behavior, the total functioning of the individual must be considered; he must feel that he is of importance as a totality, that he is more than speech alone.

Healthier personalities usually develop as better speech is achieved. However, if personalities do not become healthier and even grow more disturbed during speech therapy meetings, the number of the meetings may need to be reduced, and careful thought needs to be directed toward the many separate variables entering into the meetings with the aim of modifying those effects which negatively affect articulation training. If reduction in the number of meetings and further thought and change concerning management do not result in healthier personalities, speech therapy needs to be discontinued temporarily and perhaps even permanently, particularly if more severe emotional disturbances result from continued speech therapy sessions. Speech therapy may continue, for example, to be provided in some settings when results are minimal and when they further aggravate personality problems of individuals who are already very threatened and insecure. The insecure person feels inadequate to begin with; he may feel even more inadequate if his speech functioning is not handled or considered in the proper perspective.

The speech pathologist needs to be very aware of the impact of the speech therapy sessions on the personality of those with whom he works. When the emotional disturbance is primarily related to speech functioning, the speech pathologist has or should have the training to handle the behavior and channel all responses into constructive purposes. The very large majority of persons receiving articulation therapy do not have emotional difficulties of a general nature. Any emotional disturbance will usually be related to the speaking behavior. In those few instances in which the emotional disturbance uncovered during speech therapy involves personality dynamics which are apparently only minimally related to speech functioning, psychological handling is indicated, with concurrent speech therapy unless the response to therapy is negative, in which case speech therapy should be discontinued. The author has described (1966) with considerable detail speech therapy with a cleft palate girl who was not able to accept the inadequacies of her speech because of total feelings of inadequacy. As we worked on reduction of nasality and better production of voiceless fricatives, she withdrew more and more from therapy and outside social situations. Although chronologically and intellectually she was 13 years old, she performed at the third grade level in school and refused to achieve beyond this level, frequently looking for materials from earlier grades. She was protecting herself from further failure by her passive behavior and emotional withdrawal. She remained at the grade level which she felt she was capable of handling. Speech therapy was discontinued temporarily, despite aberrant speech, for two reasons: (1) speech training could not be approached in a manner that would result in a healthier person, and (2) speech functioning not only did not improve, but efforts to improve speech resulted in a more disturbed individual.

The speech therapy procedures which follow are suggested for different age groups. But the sensitivity toward personality dynamics involved during the therapy sessions is important for all groups.

PRESCHOOL CHILDREN

As a general rule, speech handling with this age group should primarily stress the grammatical dimension and continued development of verbal output while linguistic rules are in the process of being learned (Menyuk, 1969). Articulation therapy, when indicated for a preschool child, needs to be sensitive to his linguistic competence. Drill materials and prodecures are made a part of those language materials which are appropriate to the linguistic level.

The child is saying his first word or words at 12 to 15 months. At two years, he is beginning to learn linguistic rules necessary for the syntactic arrangement of short phrases of two and three words in length. These responses are structurally incomplete, as many words are lacking which are syntactically necessary. However, many responses are functionally complete, since the full meaning of the child's utterances may be understood when listeners supply the missing words. Responses become syntactically more structurally complete as the child becomes older, resulting in utterances of greater length. At three years of age, a child's responses average approximately three words in length; at four years of age responses average approximately four words in length; and at five and six years of age, upon entering kindergarten, the child's responses are complete structurally, averaging five to seven words in length. The linguistic rules necessary for forming structurally complete simple sentences have been learned, and rules for forming certain other kinds of sentences have been learned as well. In four years, then, the speech of the child has grown from incomplete phrases and a superficial knowledge of syntax to structurally complete simple sentences and knowledge of the linguistic rules necessary for the formation of structurally complete sentences (Goda, 1970). During the preschool years a child also repeats words, whether whole words or parts of words. Repetitions are particularly prominent when the child is excited about his verbal descriptions, with the excitement resulting in increased rate as well. Excessive repetition can also occur when a child has a considerable amount of talking to do and lacks the proper vocabulary or feels unsure of the correctness of his words.

When articulation therapy is indicated for a preschool child, the materials commensurate with the linguistic and emotional levels of the child are used. Speech is in the process of being learned as a total kind of behavior. All dimensions will be fully mastered if speech is rewarded sufficiently so that it can become self-reenforcing. As the child speaks more in a rewarding environment, he continues to speak even more because of the resultant effects of speech on persons in his environment. The child in a punitive or nonrewarding environment may speak relatively little because of the punishing effects which result from speaking.

Mowrer (1958) has elaborated this concept. He discusses the reasons why some children learn to speak while others do not. The children who learn to speak hear "good" sounds from a loving, caring mother in an environment which is totally rewarding. Applying Mowrer's principles, articulation therapy can be maximally effective with the preschool child if all elements in the environment are pleasing. Speech has not yet become a tool unto itself but exists only as a part of his total behavior and reaction system.

The speech functioning of preschool children is highly egocentric. Piaget (1955) discusses in considerable detail how they use speech as a part of their play activity. However, they do not use speech in a socialized manner as do older children and adults. As children play with fire engines or cars, language becomes an essential ingredient and almost an extension of the "car," with production of sound effects appropriate to the scenario being enacted. In such a set, children do not always welcome verbal responses from an adult listener unless the adult has become an intrinsic part of the play activity, in which case the presence and utterances of the adult become part of the entire activity. Unless the clinician is able to fit therapy activities into the play activities subtly, children may inhibit their play activity and consequently speak less.

The play behavior of the preschool child is also likely to be highly egocentric. The individual preschool child is initially a solitary player and usually a nongroup participant, preferring to play alone without being burdened by the desires and wants of someone else. While these children usually play alone, their play may be parallel, since each child plays side by side with other children but the activity of each child is separate. As they play in the same physical environment, they will direct remarks to each other but without any need for responses. The parallel play of children can be very dissimilar, similar, or even identical, but this seems to make no real difference to the child, unless someone intrudes or handles the play material in any way, in which case the child may become very angry and highly negative. Over a period of time, preschool children will learn to share possessions and play with each other, but work toward this goal must be carried on very slowly, with great concern and regard for the child and his feelings. Nursery school programs seek to develop a sharing and playing together, as must any program which deals with preschool children. Secure or mature preschool children will adapt to and learn sharing with others more quickly than less secure or immature preschool children. As a group, preschool children with speech difficulties may be less secure than children without them. If a child has difficulty making himself understood, adults in his environment will usually let it be known that he is not understood; then the child may begin to inhibit both play and speaking activities, which are usually very closely integrated as has been described. As the child reveals less and less of himself in his play-speech activities, feelings of security become reduced. While all children with speech difficulties do not feel insecure in speaking situations with adults, some have many fears and feelings of insecurity concerning speech because of the effects of their speech on the response of others. Punishing effects and an absence of positive rewards can result from their speaking. We know that unrewarded behavior becomes less and less frequent. Thus the child with a speech difficulty may tend to speak less, and will consequently have less practice in speaking.

Like any motor skill, speech needs to be practiced if the skill is to be learned. The statement often made by Dr. Wendell Johnson concerning the stutterer ("his speaking time is his working time") is equally true for the child with an articulation disturbance. If the child's speech is to improve, he needs to practice. However, he is not likely to speak more unless the environment rewards his speaking behavior. In the event that the environment does not reward speaking behavior, speech will remain at the same relatively low level or become even less.

Speech therapy procedures with the preschool child need to be fitted into a therapeutic milieu in which the emotional needs of the children are paramount. Extreme sensitivity to the child's feelings must be maintained, with recognition of the vital role of speech in interaction with persons in social situations. If the child enjoys speech, its benefits, and the persons relating socially to him, he is likely to flourish in speech therapy situations. If, however, he does not enjoy speech, derives pain from it, and dislikes persons involved in communicative situations, he will present negative withdrawal reactions to all procedures and materials involved in speech therapy. Results will obviously be very limited in view of such reactions as these.

Before speech therapy is begun with a preschool child, his spontaneous play activity should be carefully studied, with regard to the amount as well as kind of speaking utilized during play. Several toys and books of presumable interest to young children can be placed in the therapy room, and the child allowed the freedom to choose whatever objects interest him. As the child plays and talks, his responses are recorded. Voice quality and fluency pattern are noted. A valid and reliable base level of speech functioning should be determined before therapy is begun. In the manner of Templin (1957) and McCarthy (1930), 50 consecutive utterances are recorded. The following data are secured from these responses; average length of response, kinds of sentences used, percentage of intelligibility, and linguistic levels.

A reliable measure of language function can be secured from 50 consecutive responses. However, these measures may not be valid. While the child uses short responses which are three to four words in length with the clinician, he may use sentences with better linguistic functioning in another situation (Goda, 1964). Responses need to be obtained until the measures are valid. It should be remembered that these utterances provide a baseline which will indicate the status of language function before therapy begins. It is not possible to evaluate the influence of therapy unless the initial measures are accurate and valid. Articulation therapy can have negative effects on linguistic functioning, as will be discussed later, resulting in shorter responses, poorer linguistic functioning, aberrant voice quality, or stuttering. These responses, if they occur, need to be noted and proper measures taken. If linguistic dimensions are not affected negatively by articulation therapy, no change is indicated in the handling of therapy, assuming, of course, that intelligibility is improving.

If further testing of articulation is indicated, the test form presented earlier may be used with appropriate pictures. While therapy with the child with an articulation disorder is concerned with intelligibility, the grammatical dimension is also important, since the child is in the process of learning the linguistic rules for all kinds of sentences. If phonemic errors alone are stressed, without regard for the grammatic and lexical dimensions, the process of learning to speak may become dull, uninteresting, frightening, or unrewarding. In reaction to the treatment the child may restrict the amount of his speaking, thus protecting himself from criticism and feelings of failure. He learns that if utterances are fewer, the number of phonemes will be fewer also. The child can develop specific word fears, thus avoiding the use of particular words because of listener responses. The sum total of a child's reaction to overemphasis on the phonemic dimension can result in an overawareness of auditory feedback. Preschool children may slow down their rate of speaking. Faulty emphasis or struggling and strained speech may also result. Bloodstein (1958, pages 31–32) describes how stuttering may develop from unreasonable and improper efforts to improve the articulation of a young child. "Stuttering at its outset is what a child does on the assumption that he will not be able to say the word without hesitating on it, mispronouncing it, misarticulating its most conspicuous sounds, saying it too rapidly or failing on it any other way." Bloodstein states further (page 36) that ". . . not hesitancy alone but anything at all which tends to shake a child's faith in his ability to speak may result in an appreciable danger that stuttering will arise sooner or later."

The speech of the preschool child is highly vulnerable because he is in the process of mastering all dimensions. Thus while one dimension may receive primary emphasis, all dimensions of speech learning must be considered as well. The listener reaction is of extreme importance. The clinician needs to be very sure that all responses to linguistic behavior will be rewarding and reenforcing. Rewards must be considered separately for each individual child; what is pleasurable and rewarding for one youngster may not be pleasurable and rewarding to another. One child might like chocolate candy excessively, and another might have severe allergy reactions to it. A child's likes and dislikes must be explored very carefully before a system for rewarding speech behavior can be developed. The child should be allowed freedom during the initial meetings to play and explore. The adult is to establish a warm comfortable environment in which all elements are pleasurable. Then speech will also become pleasurable, because it is intricately involved with the total environment. As we have said, preschool children do not use speech as an isolated tool as do adults or older children; rather, their speech is involved intimately in their physical play activities. If the toys provide fun, the adult applauds the fun; if speech related to the play is fun, the child will begin to use speech easily and naturally. The adult initially needs to be able to feed back to the child the responses he has had to the play material. As the child makes the appropriate noises with cars, guns, and airplanes, the adult needs to imitate these sounds. Obviously the child can begin to feel comfortable with the adult if his sound making is the same as the child's. As the adult imitates the speech and play of the child more and more, the immediate relationship between the two will gradually become deeper and more involved. The child will begin to enjoy and accept the presence and involvement of the adult. The adult can gradually introduce speech which is appropriate to the play. The child will either imitate the responses of the adult or may continue his own verbal responses. Cars can crash with sirens whistling, people screaming; guns can fire with bodies falling and horses galloping, etc. Speech associated with these activities will initially provide sound effects, with slight regard for propositional speech as such.

As the adult and child become secure with each other, appropriate propositional speech can be introduced. The toys may not be visible, and the child may have to request a particular toy. The adult may now express pleasure at the choice as the toy is taken out; he may ask the reason for the preference. As scenes develop, speech is introduced naturally by the adult if the child has not already done so. They talk about what they have done in their play behavior together. They talk about what has happened and what will happen. The clinician and child are in essence making a game of speech. They imitate each other and use speech as part of play activities. Further, the child needs to be allowed to engage in soliloquies without interruption from the adult, who listens and records the speech of the child during these soliloquies. These two activities, imitation and soliloquy, have been noted to be examples "of children's tendency to play with skills at their disposal" (McNeill, 1966, page 72).

The phonemic dimensions can be considered very briefly, by the isolation of words out of a context in which they have been spoken incorrectly because of consonant errors. The phonemes selected should be those which are very frequently produced correctly in some phonetic context, and which are among the sounds that, according to various studies, the preschool child produces correctly. Plosives can be considered initially. The child might remark, "Put the car up here." The /p/ in releasing the word *put* might be produced correctly, but the consonant might be omitted in arresting the word *up*. Usually the child will include the sound if the adult says the word several times and instructs him to imitate production of the word. Now the word *up* can be used very frequently in play activity, as the adult seeks a situation in which the word might be included. You might have the child *come up, go up, look up*, and *stand up*. The adult might do these things as well as part of the play activity. As they discuss what has happened, both the child and adult will seek to use the word frequently. Another instance of plosive error inconsistency might be revealed as the child remarks, "I come back now," with correct production of /k/ in *come* but omission in *back*. The word *back* can be isolated and used as was done with *up*. When you return from any activity you are *back*, the lost toy is *back*, and finally at the end of the lesson the word can be used very meaningfully in stating "I will be back tomorrow."

Other words may be chosen, but it is important that the play activity be the important pursuit, with speech enriching the play activity. Any articulation training should be done very briefly without disturbing the play activity or meaningful speech associated with the play. The lexical and grammatical dimensions are rewarded by the effects of the global speech behavior on the play.

As speech becomes more and more useful in play, speech can now be isolated from play and become a part of reading activities. Preschool children listen very well to stories and can become quite involved in the activities of persons and animals involved in the stories. The adult can skillfully interrupt the story at a particular point for articulation training, but the integrity of the story should not be disturbed. Articulation training while necessary and important is of less importance to the child than completion of the story.

As an example, the author was working with a four-year-old child who had inconsistent errors involving the velar plosives /k/ and /g/. The story read to him was *Will You Come to My Party?* (Asheron, 1961). The squirrel asks each animal "Will you come to my party?" At the beginning, the two of us together issued the invitation but later the child did the inviting alone. The animals in the *garden* who were invited were the *cat* and the *dog*. The squirrel had nuts in the *basket* for all the animals. The rabbit wanted *carrots. Carrots* would be *good* for him, but nuts in the *basket* would not be *good*. Squirrel *begins* to *cry because* he has no *carrots*. He *talks* to the bird. He *talks* to the rabbit. He *talks* to the *girl* and boy, etc. The story can be read several times, and also it may be recalled.

Finally speech can be used judiciously in discussing the feelings of the young preschool child. Before we read the story one day, the author noted that the child was limping. He had trouble *walking*. He *could* not *walk good*.

His *leg* hurt. His *leg* hurt when he would *walk*. He did not *like* to be in pain. He wished his *leg* would *become O.K. again.*

Many preschool children produce consonants correctly to release the syllable but omit the sound in arresting the syllable. Errors of omission have been mentioned as the principal type of error among preschool children (Milisen, 1954). Errors of omission can be corrected relatively easily, particularly if the sound has already been produced correctly in some phonetic context, since there will now be only one task to learn or discrimination to make: that of including the sound consistently. Usually several phonemic errors of omission can be handled simultaneously, as the goal is the teaching of sound production in all contexts. Once the child begins including a single sound, he will then usually begin to include other sounds, particularly if the other sounds have been involved in training. For example, the child who begins to include /g/ in *dog* will have a very easy time with the process of including other plosives to arrest syllables.

EARLY ELEMENTARY SCHOOL AGE CHILDREN

Children in the early elementary grades are beginning to use speech as a tool, but the function of speech is still largely egocentric. Thus while therapy can involve some speech tasks without involvement in any play activity, some time needs to be allowed for play and speech associated with play. Play activity of this age child will be richer and more involved than that of the preschool child. Whereas the preschool child might end the scene after a few minutes of play with very few characters involved, the child in the first and second grades will have very involved stories with many different characters. As with the preschool child, words can be taken out of context for quick drill purposes. Thorough articulation testing in the manner described previously should be done before therapy is started.

Whenever possible drill words should come from the child's experiences and desires. For example, a first grade child learning to write was writing the letter "h." As he was writing and saying the name of the letter, he referred to the letter name as the diphthong /eɪ/ omitting /tʃ/.

He was interested in saying the correct name for the letters because this was important in school. Thus he said the letter name continuously until production was correct. One child eager to discuss the *marriage* of his *cousin* distorted nasals. His speech was hyponasal with distortions of all nasal consonants, but there was no physical basis for the errors. We talked about the *marriage*, the *many* people who would *come*, the dress his *mother* would wear, the *names* of the bride and *groom*, the *minister*, the *time* they would leave *home*, when they would *come* up the aisle, the *music* they would play, the *songs* they would *sing*, the *ring* he would put on her *finger*, his *new cousins* he *had not met* yet, etc. The event was the important item, and so it was important at least initially that the content and feelings of the event be revealed. Words were isolated with the view of not disturbing the discussion per se. The initial narration was told with only several interruptions. The event was described again with a few more interruptions. Both of us were now involved in the telling, I providing some personal experiences of weddings attended. Finally words were taken out of context and drilled until production was correct. The tape recorder was used to point out the differences between my productions and his, and those of his productions which were correct and those which were incorrect.

Many instances of articulation errors are related to word length. Children might produce /k/ in *key* but omit it in *monkey, turkey, donkey*. Fractionation of the words into the two syllables can bring quick results. Frequently errors involving a single consonant can be corrected by contrasting word lists involving the consonant as a single and in blends. Correction of a /l/ distortion occurred rather quickly using this approach. The words *clean, clues, clock, clay, clamp* in which the /l/ was produced correctly were compared with *lean, lose, lock, lay,* and *lamp* in which the phoneme was produced incorrectly. (See blend contrast lists, Chapter 3, for a more extensive list.)

If the child can read the words for drills, the lists should be written. If he is not a reader, pictures should be used, and he may imitate production, or a combination of reading and repeating may be utilized.

The sounds chosen for first handling will be those in which production is already correct in some phonetic contexts. Sounds not produced correctly in any phonetic context are viewed with the aim of selecting, in the beginning, those sounds which are produced correctly in some phonetic context following stimulation. The remaining errors will involve consonants which are not produced correctly following stimulation. From those sounds, the ones chosen first will be those which are produced correctly in some phonetic context embedded in nonsense syllables. If sounds remain which are not produced correctly in nonsense syllables, the ones chosen at first will be those which are produced the most nearly correct, with training involving gradual shaping until production is correct. The phonetic contexts resulting in successful or near-successful productions, as the case may be, provide the material for articulation training in the manner described previously. Games may be played to motivate the child or as a reward. However, as mentioned before, it is important that games not be an end to themselves but that they serve as the means of securing better results in speech training. Quicker results can probably be secured from most children if game playing is discarded or minimized very early in speech training.

Error hierarchy will also furnish a basis for sound selection. Developmentally, as has been discussed, the omission error is at the lowest level and the distortion error is at the highest level. The preschool child is not aware of the significance of, distinctions between, and necessity for all sounds, and so he omits many. When the child is in school, he may be aware of the importance of all sounds but cannot produce them all successfully. He can approximate the correct production but may not produce the sound exactly correctly, resulting in a substandard and unacceptable production of the target sound. However, the omission error will usually be corrected the most easily, as the teaching involves the learning and production of one sound only. The child has only one discrimination to learn. The child who distorts the sound, however, has at least two discriminations to learn. He must replace his incorrect production with the correct one. The child with the substitution error has at least two discrimination tasks to learn also. For example, the child might substitute /t/ for /k/. He will need to learn those words in which /t/ is the correct phoneme and those in which /k/ is the correct phoneme. He must learn to produce the /k/ sound when necessary phonemically, and he must retain production of /t/ when necessary phonemically. It may happen that the child might distort the omitted sound when he attempts production. Under these circumstances, errors of distortion, if there are any, should be considered before the omission error.

OLDER CHILDREN AND ADULTS

When the child has reached third grade or beyond he is using speech as a tool for communication of ideas. He is reading and learning more about the world as a result. Articulation drills can now be practiced without many efforts being required for making the procedure more palatable through games.

Discussions of feelings are particularly important with older children and adults. While they are likely to be more highly motivated than younger children because they know the importance of good speech, they are also likely to be highly embarrassed and ashamed, particularly if they have been receiving therapy for any length of time, and if they feel they do not have support from their environment.

If encouraged to express these feelings, they will usually be more strongly motivated, especially if progress is continuous and apparent. While acquaintances and perhaps even friends may not provide emotional support, the warmth, manners, and kindness of the clinician may well provide the support which is needed until the phonemic dimension of speech is mastered fully. Parents can also provide children with the necessary emotional support; this will be discussed later.

Adolescents are particularly sensitive about speech difficulty because they are beginning to be involved in dating and social functions. Poor speech can be a great deterrent to social popularity. Good speech can enhance opportunities for greater social popularity. Adults seeking new jobs or advancement can either be hindered by poor speech or assisted by good speech. Both the adolescent and the adult will need a speech pathologist with whom they can discuss their feelings. They will feel that their speech cannot be of much significance to the clinician if they are not allowed the freedom to discuss those areas which are of the most importance.

INDIVIDUAL THERAPY VERSUS GROUP THERAPY

In many instances, group therapy can be utilized because of the large numbers of persons in need of speech therapy compared with the small number of speech clinicians available. However, when a choice can be made, it should be determined by the needs of the individual who is in need of therapy.

Some individuals achieve better results when involved in a group, while others achieve results only when seen individually. For example, adolescents often function better in a group setting because they learn more from each other than from an adult. However, the adolescent who is highly self-conscious and fearful of group participation should be seen individually until he can learn to adapt to others without fear of losing his identity. As another example, preschool children should be seen individually because of their egocentricity in speech function and play. Further, remembering the disastrous results which can occur as a result of articulation training, the clinician has to be focused on and highly sensitive to the impact of therapy on the speech functioning of a child. Sensitivity and proper handling can best be achieved if the clinician sees one child at a time.

Some individuals cannot adapt to group behavior because they wish to maintain their individuality. Some adults, for example, might be quite disturbed by being placed in a group with others who have similar speech problems. They insist that their problem is unlike that of anyone else, and while the logic of this might be argued the effect of this kind of thinking on therapeutic results is the crucial issue. If individual therapy produces significant results and group placement results in unproductive, negative behavior, therapy needs to be conducted on an individual basis. Many so-called autistic children can function only in a one-to-one situation because of emotional fears when involved in activities of others. Individual treatment with these children is mandatory if beneficial results are to occur from speech therapy.

LENGTH AND FREQUENCY OF SPEECH THERAPY SESSIONS

All things being equal, the child with the most severe speech problem is in need of the most intensive treatment. However, the age, motivation, and emotional maturity of the child all need to be considered in any planning. The status of the family and the emotional feelings of the mother need to be considered also, with care taken not to aggravate guilt feelings of the mother. Realistic requirements need to be placed on the mother, but with regard for her other involvements and the needs of the other family members. For example, a mother with other children of school age may have considerable difficulty in keeping more than one appointment per week. When illness occurs in the family, she may well have difficulty in keeping even the single weekly appointment.

The length and frequency of the meetings are not as important as what occurs during the meetings. Many children may well work for the fully allotted time of half an hour or even an hour. Other children are not able to sustain the effort for a full period. Fully as much (if not more) learning may occur during a five-minute segment as during a thirty-minute segment. The feelings of the defective speaker and his involvement in speech learning are the crucial issues. Nothing should occur during the meetings to make speech learning painful or laborious. Rather, if at all possible, speech learning should fit naturally and comfortably into a social situation involving the group and clinician in the group situation and an individual and clinician in an individual situation.

PARENTAL INVOLVEMENT

Many programs unwisely seek to involve the parent in articulation training, ostensibly because the child spends many more hours at home than in school. Some research even indicates that articulation results are significantly better if the parent has some training in articulation management (Sommers et al., 1958), reviving a thought of many years ago ("Make mother a clinician," Lillywhite, 1948).

If we make mother a clinician, the reading teacher might want to make her a reading teacher, the math teacher might want her to teach math, and the nurse might even want her to be a health teacher. With such a regimen, there would not be very much time for the mother to be a parent, which is a highly demanding and involved job. The mother who provides the best support for her child in all learning activities is the mother who provides the environment necessary for the learning of tasks. One can only pity the poor child who faces speech therapy in school and then must face it again in his own home, where his mother may previously have been accepting and understanding, but now is as critical and demanding as school. We could make stutterers of all children with articulation disorders if parents become highly critical and demanding of articulation mastery.

Even if speech results may be somewhat better when the parent becomes involved, imagine the effect on the parent-child relationship! Spontaneity between parent and child becomes impossible when a parent is teaching as well as providing love. Wood (1946) reports on the maladjustment of parents of children with articulation disorders. Obviously such parents should not be involved in corrective training at home.

If our aim is articulation mastery alone, then factors which enhance articulation development should be our sole consideration. But if we are involved in the emotional development of the children, then we must investigate many more factors before we involve the average parent in speech therapy. Most of us lack the time and facilities for thorough exploration of the parent, the parent's reaction to the child, and vice versa. Speech pathologists have the responsibility of correcting speech disorders. They evade responsibility by turning the task over to persons who are untrained. The parent-child relationship needs to be understood and supported. Its structure might be weakened considerably if too many demands are placed on the relationship.

Developmental studies of children previously mentioned indicate that articulation is not mastered before the age of eight years, and that children in the first and second grades may be expected to have articulation errors. As children become older, their articulation naturally improves with practice. This practice is best provided in a home environment which offers valuable support and encouragement for intellectual, emotional, and social development. The mother who is warm and spontaneous can provide this support. The child who is slower in his articulation development may well need the speech therapy which is offered now in hospital, school, or private settings. The professional management offered, together with valuable emotional support from the home, can provide easy management for the child's problem. However, the parent who becomes a teacher must become critical, and thus the natural spontaneity and warmth of the parent is curtailed. Over a period of time, this kind of parental involvement can lead to more harm than good. Increased anxiety may be reflected in a strained parent-child relationship. In some few instances where the problem is particularly severe and not amenable to speech therapy because of personal factors, help from the parent may be necessary. Before requesting parental help, however, the parent-child relationship needs careful exploration. If this exploration indicates that the relationship is strong, good, secure, and comfortable, greater requirements may be placed on it within narrowly prescribed limits and with periodic reevaluation of the relationship with the passing of time.

References

Asheron, Sara A.: Will You Come to My Party? New York, Wonder Books, 1961.

Baratz, Joan C.: Language and cognitive assessment of Negro children: assumptions and research needs. ASHA 11:87–91, 1969.

Berry, Mildred F., and Eisenson, J.: Speech Disorders: Principles and Practice of Therapy. New York, Appleton-Century-Crofts, 1956.

Black, J.: The pressure component in the production of consonants. J. Speech Hearing Dis. 15:207–210, 1950.

Bloodstein, O.: Stuttering as an anticipatory struggle reaction. In: Eisenson, J.: Stuttering, a Symposium. New York, Harper & Bros., 1958.

Curtis, J., and Hardy, J.: A phonetic study of misarticulation of /r/. J. Speech Hearing Res. 2:244–257, 1959.

Developmental Articulation Test. Madison, Wis., College Typing Co., 1959.

Fairbanks, G.: Voice and Articulation Drillbook (ed. 2). New York, Harper & Bros., 1960.

Fries, C. C.: The Structure of English. New York, Harcourt, Brace & Co., 1952.

————: Linguistics and Reading. New York, Holt, Rinehart & Winston, 1963.

Garrett, E. R.: Discussant, ASHA Section, Meeting of AAAS. ASHA, 10:203–204, 1968.

Gleason, H. A.: An Introduction to Descriptive Linguistics. New York, Holt, Rinehart & Winston, 1961.

Goda, S.: Comment on temporal reliability of seven language measures. J. Speech Hearing Res. 7:298, 1964.

————: Speech therapy with selected patients with congenital velopharyngeal inadequacy. Cleft Palate J. 3:268–274, 1966.

————: The role of the speech pathologist in the correction of tongue-thrust. Amer. J. Orthodont. 54:852–859, 1968.

————: Speech development of children. Amer. J. Nurs. 70:276–279, 1970.

Hockett, C. F.: A Course in Modern Linguistics. New York, Macmillan, 1958.

Holland, Audrey L.: Some applications of behavioral principles to clinical speech problems. J. Speech Hearing Dis. 32:11–18, 1967.

Irwin, O. C.: Infant speech: consonantal sounds according to manner of articulation. J. Speech Dis. 12:397–401, 1947A.

————: Infant speech: consonantal sounds according to manner of articulation. J. Speech Dis. 12:402–404, 1947B.

Johnson, W., Brown, S. F., Curtis, J. F., Edney, C. W., and Keaster, Jacqueline: Speech Handicapped School Children (ed. 3). New York, Harper & Bros., 1967.

Kenyon, J. S., and Knott, T. A.: A Pronouncing Dictionary of American English. Springfield, Mass., G. & C. Merriam, 1944.

Lewis, M. M.: Infant Speech: A Study of the Beginnings of Language. New York, Humanities Press, 1951.

Lillywhite, H.: Make mother a clinician. J. Speech Hearing Dis. 13:61–66, 1948.

McCarthy, Dorothea E.: The Language Development of the Pre-School Child. Minneapolis, University of Minnesota Press, 1930.

McDonald, E. T.: Articulation Testing and Treatment: A Sensory Motor Approach. Pittsburgh, Stanwix House, 1964A.

———: A Deep Test of Articulation, Picture Form. Pittsburgh, Stanwix House, 1964B.

———: A Deep Test of Articulation, Sentence Form. Pittsburgh, Stanwix House, 1964C.

McNeill, D.: Developmental psycholinguistics. In: The Genesis of Language. Cambridge, Mass., M.I.T. Press, 1966.

Menyuk, Paula: Sentences Children Use. Cambridge, Mass. M.I.T. Press, 1969.

Milisen, R. L.: The disorder of articulation: a systematic clinical and experimental approach. J. Speech Hearing Dis. Supplement, 1954.

Mowrer, O.: Speech development in the young child: the autism theory of speech development and some clinical applications. J. Speech Hearing Dis. 17:263–268, 1958.

Olson, W.: Child Development (ed. 2). Boston, D. C. Heath, 1959.

Piaget, J.: The Language and Thought of the Child. New York, Meridian Books, 1955.

Powers, Margaret H.: Functional disorders of articulation—symptomatology and etiology. In: Travis, L. (Ed.): Handbook of Speech Pathology. New York, Appleton-Century-Crofts, 1957, pp. 707–768.

Roe, Vivian, and Milisen, R. L.: Effect of maturation upon defective articulation in elementary grades. J. Speech Dis. 7:37–50, 1942.

Schoolfield, Lucille: Better Speech and Better Reading. Boston, Expression Co., 1951.

Shohara, H.: Significance of overlapping movements in speech. In: McDonald, E. T.: Articulation Testing and Treatment, a Sensory Motor Approach, 1964, pp. 19–27.

Sommers, R. K., Shilling, S. P., Paul, Clara D., Copetas, Florence G., Bowser, Dolores C., and McClintock, Colette J.: Training parents of children with functional misarticulation. J. Speech Hearing Res. 2:258–265, 1958.

Spriestersbach, D. C., and Curtis, J. F.: Misarticulation and discrimination of speech sounds. Quart. J. Speech 37:483–491, 1951.

Spriestersbach, D. C., Moll, K. L., and Morris, H. L.: Subject classification and articulation of speakers with cleft palate. J. Speech Hearing Res. 4:362–372, 1961.

Spriestersbach, D. C., and Powers, G. R.: Articulation skills, velopharyngeal closure and oral breath pressure of children with cleft palates. J. Speech Hearing Res. 2:318–325, 1959.

Stetson, R. H.: (1951). Motor Phonetics. Amsterdam, North Holland Publishing Co., 1951.

Templin, Mildred C.: Spontaneous versus imitated verbalization in testing articulation in preschool children. J. Speech Dis. 12:293–300, 1947.

———: Certain Language Skills in Children, Institute of Child Welfare Monograph Series 26. Minneapolis, University of Minnesota Press, 1957.

Templin, Mildred C., and Darley, F.: The Templin-Darley Tests of Articulation. Iowa City, Iowa, University of Iowa, 1960.

Thorndike, E. S., and Lorge, I.: The Teacher's Word Book of 30,000 Words. New York, Columbia University Press, 1944.

Van Riper, C. V.: Speech Correction, Principles and Methods (ed. 4). Englewood Cliffs, N.J., Prentice-Hall, 1965.

Van Riper, C. V., and Irwin, J. V.: Voice and Articulation. Englewood Cliffs, N.J., Prentice-Hall, 1958.

Williams, D.: A point of view about stuttering. J. Speech Hearing Dis. 22:390–397, 1957.

Winitz, H.: The development of speech and language in the normal child. In: Rieber, R. W., and Brubaker, R. S.: Speech Pathology: An International Study of the Science. Amsterdam, North Holland Publishing Co., 1966, pp. 42–76.

Wood, K. S.: Parental maladjustment and functional articulatory defects in children. J. Speech Hearing Dis. 11:255–275, 1946.

Index

Adaptation of speech therapy to age
  adults, 143, 153, 154
  preschool, 143, 144–151, 153
  school age, 143, 151–154
Allomorphs, 117
Allophones, 11, 127
Appliance to control tongue placement, 138
Articulation disorder
  evaluation, 102, 108, 139, 151
    movement sequences, 105
    by position, 105, 106
    whole word method, 113, 117, 118–126
  treatment, 60, 102, 104, 115, 116, 143–145, 147, 150, 151
    movement sequences, 110–113
    stimulation method, 105, 106, 108, 111, 113
    whole word method, 113, 117, 126–136
Asheron, Sara A., 150
Auditory confusion, 90
  drill materials, 97–99
Auditory discrimination, viii, 106, 109, 132
Auditory modality, 132, 141

Baratz, Joan C., 117
Basis of articulation disorder
  functional etiology, vii, ix, 1, 138
  organic etiology, vii, 1, 138, 151
    aphasia, vii
    cerebral palsy, vii
    cleft palate, vii, 127, 144
    dysarthria, viii
    mental retardation, vii
Berry, Mildred F., 2
Black, J., 130
Blends, 2, 4, 84, 90, 102, 103, 107, 115, 116, 119, 121, 123, 125, 126, 134, 135, 139, 140, 152

drill material for three-element blends, 78, 79
drill material for two-element blends, 66–78, 80–83, 100, 101
  /d/ blends, 82, 83
  [l] blends, 66–69
  [r] blends, 70–75
  /s/ blends, 75–78
  /t/ blends, 80–82
  /w/ blends, 83
  See also Articulation disorder; Whole word method, blend production
Bloodstein, O., 148
Breath pressure
  inadequacy with cleft palate speakers, 130
  need for, 137
Breath stream, viii, 2, 3, 4, 11, 13, 14, 20, 34, 41, 56, 84, 125, 136, 141

Carrier phrases, 9
Carry-over, 106
Caseload, viii, 1
Child development, 114
Compensation, 135
Connected speech, 5
Connective words, 9, 10, 129, 132
Consistent articulation errors, 141, 142
Consonant classification
  function of consonant, 127
    arresting of syllable, 2, 3, 5, 13–15, 17–19, 22, 25, 28, 30, 32, 34, 37, 42, 44, 47–49, 51, 53, 56, 58, 66, 75–77, 80–84, 112, 117, 120, 122–131, 151
    releasing of syllable, 2, 3, 5, 13–15, 16, 18, 19, 22–24, 26–28, 31–39, 42, 43, 45–48, 50–52, 54, 55, 57–62, 66–79, 83, 84, 112, 117, 120–131, 139, 140, 151

159

placement, 12, 13, 90, 127
  drill materials, 95, 96
positional, 2, 60, 102, 104, 105
  final position, 63–65, 102, 118, 119, 124
  initial position, 62, 102, 115, 118, 119, 124
  medial position, 63, 64, 102, 118, 119
voicing, 12, 127, 131
  drill materials, vii, 1, 12, 13, 20, 24, 29, 33, 41, 46, 53, 59
  voiced sounds, 12, 20, 41, 56, 90
  voiceless sounds, 12, 20, 41, 56, 80, 144
Consonant errors
  consistency of error, vii, 103, 104, 108–110, 112, 113, 115, 116, 119, 121, 125, 133–135, 138, 139, 143, 150
  types of errors, 102
    distortions, 90, 102–104, 112, 117–119, 125, 127, 135–138, 151, 153
    omissions, 60, 102–104, 109, 116–119, 128, 150, 151, 153
    substitutions, 60, 102–104, 109, 114, 117–119, 153
Consonant types
  affricates or combinations, 2, 9, 12, 56, 87, 88, 115, 119, 125, 136
    drill materials for, 56–59
  fricatives, 2, 9, 12, 34, 41, 56, 86, 87, 114–116, 119, 125, 130, 131, 133, 135–137, 144
    drill materials for, 41–55
  glides, 2, 11, 34, 60, 90, 119, 125, 133, 139
  nasals, 2, 11, 14, 34, 84, 119, 125, 151
    drill materials for ,14–19
  plosives, 2, 8, 12, 20, 34, 56, 85, 86, 90, 128, 130, 131, 135–137, 140, 149–151
    drill materials for, 20–33, 91–94
  semivowels, 2, 11, 34, 88, 119, 132, 135, 136
    drill materials for, 35–40
Continuants, 41, 130
Contrast lists, 1, 12, 13, 41, 56
  drill materials, 91–101
  voicing contrasts. See Consonant classification, voicing
Cross-sectional study, 114
Curtis, J., 2, 4, 60, 109, 138, 139
Cutting edge, 135

Darley, F., 102, 103, 105
Different /l/ sounds, 2, 11, 34, 38–40, 134–136
Different /r/ sounds
  consonant glide [r], 2, 11, 60–62, 133, 138, 139
  drill materials for, 60–65
  intervocalic [r], 60, 138
  stressed vocalic [ɝ], 2, 11, 60, 62, 63, 138–140
  unstressed vocalic [ɚ], 2, 11, 60, 64, 138, 140
Diphthongs, 2, 103, 151
Discussion of feelings, 150, 153, 154
Discussion topics, 8, 9, 121, 149
"Do" language, 126
Duration, 137

Ear training, 106, 109
Earliest learned sounds, 2, 13
Ease of articulation, 124
Eclectic approach, ix
Egocentric speech, 146, 151, 154
Eisenson, J., 2
Emotional disturbance and relation to articulation disorder, 144
Emotional feelings during therapy
  anxiety, 143
  impact of speech therapy, 112, 144, 148, 149, 154
  trust and respect, 143
Error hierarchy, 153

Fairbanks, G., 2, 11, 34, 60, 105, 136
Feedback systems
  auditory, 106, 108, 109, 110, 116, 117, 126, 148
  kinesthetic, 106, 126
  proprioceptive, 110
  tactual, 106, 110, 126
Feelings of guilt, 155
Flexibility of consonant function, 5, 130, 131
Fractionation of words, 152
Frequency of sound, 126
Fries, C. C., 6
Function words, 6, 129

Games, 106–108, 152, 153
Garrett, E. R., 138
Gleason, H. A., 11, 41, 111

Goda, S., 116, 137, 144, 145, 147
Grammatical dimensions
    isolated word level, vii, 5, 6, 13, 113, 114,
        127
    kinds of sentences, 147
    phrases of varying length, vii, 6–9, 113,
        114, 130
    structurally complete simple sentence,
        vii, 9, 13
    syntax, 6, 145
Group therapy, 154

Hardy, J., 2, 4, 60, 138, 139
Hockett, C. F., 11
Holland, Audrey L., 109

Imitation of speech, 149, 150
Individual therapy, 154
Integral stimulation
    procedure in, 121, 123
    testing of effects of, on consonants as
        singles, 122
        on two- and three-element blends, 173
        on vocalic [r] and vocalic [l], 123
    use of, 123, 124, 125
Intelligibility, 116, 126, 138, 147, 148
Intensity, 137
Interdental tongue placement, 133, 134,
    136, 137
Irwin, J. V., 2, 106
Irwin, O. C., 114

Johnson, W., 2, 11, 106, 126, 147

Kenyon, J. S., 60
Knott, T. A., 60

Latest learned sounds, 2, 13
Level for beginning articulation therapy
    auditory discrimination level, 124
    nonsense syllable level, 124, 125, 141
    word level, 124, 125
Lewis, M. M., 114
Lexicon, 1, 148, 150
Lillywhite, H., 155
Limitations of tests of articulation, 103–
    105
Linguistics
    competence in, 144
    efficiency in, 117

linguistic level, 144, 145, 147
    first word or words, 145
    linguistic rules, 144, 145, 148
    See also Grammatical dimensions
Lip occlusion, 134
Lip rounding, 132, 133, 135, 141
Lip spreading, 132, 133, 141
Lisp, 11
Longer speech units, 132
Lorge, I., vii, 1, 90

Mastery of consonant phonemes, 1, 2, 113,
    115, 153, 156
McCarthy, Dorothea E., 147
McDonald, E. T., 2, 104, 105, 111, 131
McNeill, D., 149
Measures of language function
    average length of response, 147
    reliable measure, 147
    valid measure, 147
Menyuk, Paula, 144
Milisen, R. L., 12, 115, 121, 151
Minimal placement requirements, 135
Misarticulation of /r/, 138–140
Morphemes, 5, 6, 117, 130
Motivation, 103, 112, 113, 121, 124, 136,
    142, 152, 153
Mowrer, O., 145
Multiple articulation errors, 133
Multiple function consonants and multiple
    blends, 84
    drill materials for consonants, 84–88
    drill materials for multiple blends, 89

Neuromuscular disorders, 105
Nursery school programs, 146

Olson, W., viii, 115
Open bite, 136
Oral reading, use of, 150
Orthodontic treatment, 136, 137
Overlapping sounds, 110

Parent-child relationship, 156
Parental involvement, 142, 153, 155
Phonetic contexts, 110, 116, 121, 123, 127,
    129, 133, 136, 138, 139, 141, 151,
    152
Piaget, J., 146
Pitch, 137
Plurals, 117, 130

Powers, G. R., 130
Powers, Margaret, 109
Prepositional phrases, 7
Programming, 109, 110
Progressive approximation, 109
Pronunciation errors, 116, 117
Psychological reactions, 121

Questions during testing, use of, 103, 121

Rate of growth, 115
Rate of speech, 5, 127, 145, 148
Reading, viii, 140, 150, 153
Relationship, 112
Repetition of words, 145
Research, ix, 155
Reward, 110, 127, 145, 146, 148
Roe, Vivian, 12, 115

Schoolfield, Lucille, 2
Schwa, 129
Sequence in language arts, viii
Shohara, H., 111, 112
Size of mouth opening, 134, 141
Soliloquy, 149
Sommers, R. K., 155
Sound, in drill words, 106, 109, 128, 150, 151
  in isolation, 106, 109, 123, 129, 130, 139, 141
  in nonsense syllable, 106, 113, 123, 141, 142, 152
Speech in play, 149–151
Spriestersbach, D. C., 109, 130
Stetson, R. H., 25, 109, 111, 123
Stress, 117, 127, 140
Stuttering, 10, 126, 147, 148, 156
Syllable division, 4, 5

Tape recorder, 152
Templin, Mildred C., 2, 11, 34, 102, 103, 105, 114, 120, 147
Terminal age, 114, 115, 156
Tests of articulation
  Deep Test of Articulation, 104, 105, 124
  Developmental Articulation Test, 102, 119

Fairbanks tests, 105
  Templin-Darley Tests, 102, 103, 105, 119
Thorndike, E. S., vii, 1, 90
Thyroid notch, 132
Tongue elevation, 14, 34, 90, 125, 132, 134–137
Tongue thrust, 137

Visibility of phonemes, 125
Voice quality
  aberrant voice quality, 148
  harshness, 10
  hoarseness, 10
  hypernasality, 10, 134, 144
  hyponasality, 151
  pleasant voice, 10
Vowels, 2, 34, 60, 103, 128, 129, 131, 133, 134, 139–141
  See also Articulation disorder; Whole word method, vowel shaping

Waiting lists, viii, 108
Whole word method, 113, 117, 118–136
  evaluation, of consonants, as singles, 118
    in three-element blends, 120
    in two-element blends, 120
    of vocalic [r] and vocalic [l], 119
  treatment, blend production, 127, 134, 135
    consonant function, 127–131
    length of word, 127, 132, 133, 139, 152
    placement, 127, 135–137
    rate, 127, 137, 138
    stress, 127, 137, 138
    voicing, 127, 131, 132
    vowel shaping, 127, 133, 134
Williams, D., 126
Winitz, H., 1
Wood, K. S., 156
Word fears, 148
Word length
  effect of on articulation, 127
  one-syllable words, vii, 3, 113, 124, 125, 129, 132, 136, 138
  polysyllabic words, vii, 3, 125, 133
  See also Articulation disorder; Whole word method, length of word